I0845503

One easy life :

My homemade salts

Éditeur:
Mathis DAURIAT
34470 Pérols

ISBN : 9798359306928
Legal Deposit : Octobre 2022
Print on demand by Amazon

Disclaimer :

This book is a practical cooking guide dedicated to anyone wishing to make homemade table salts to delight friends and family.

Disclaimer

Eat salt but not too much!

In the United States, the salt consumption is about 15 g per day, but the World Health Organization (WHO) recommends barely 5 g per day, or half!

But don't forget that 80% of the salt we consume is hidden in the foods we eat every day.

Consuming iodized salt is highly recommended to prevent iodine deficiency

Introduction

Homemade table salts, that's a change !

The objective of this book is not to encourage you to consume more salt but the opposite. With varying salts, you will learn to consume less salt and discover new flavors that salt coupled with spices can offer!

Not to mention that spices are rich in antioxidants and have many health benefits!

What are you waiting for to prepare your homemade salts?

Benefits and harms of salt

Strengths as well as faults!

Health benefits of salt

Salt is the main mineral component of blood and extracellular fluids in the body. It plays a very important role in maintaining our overall health.

Here are some benefits of salt:

- in the transmission of impulses in nerve and muscle tissue
- Contributes to the maintenance of the balance between the various liquids of the body
- Improves the hydration of our cells
- Regulates acid-base balance
- Increases appetite *(flavor enhancer)*

• Increases the speed of recovery for athletes. It compensates for the loss of salt due to sweating.

The dangers of excess salt

Excess salt causes the following harms:

• Aggravates water rétention phenomena

• Increase in blood pressure which can lead to high blood pressure

• Increases the risk of osteoporosis *(decreased bone density)* and kidney stones

• Disrupts the intestinal microbiota by creating a decrease in the rate of lactobacillus *(bacteria essential to the intestinal flora)*

• Increases the risk of headaches *(headaches)* in hypertensive patients

Some numbers

• 300 to 400,000 vascular accidents every year in France

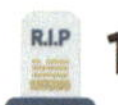 150,000 people die...

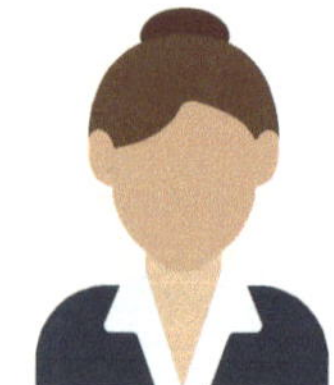

Average consumption

8,2g/day   10,2g/day

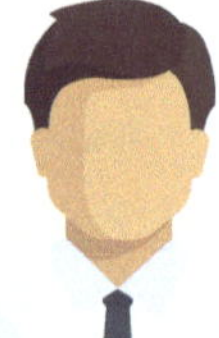

• Production d'environ 295 Production of around 295 million tonnes of salt per year worldwide

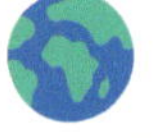 About 9.3 tons of salt every second

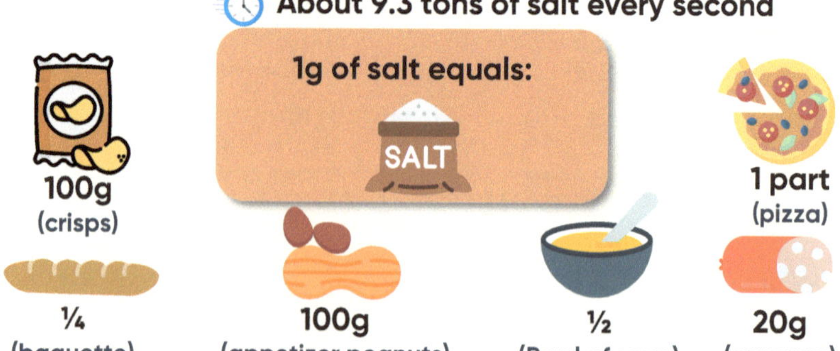

How the book works

This book is composed of 2 different summaries.

The first is the summary by nomenclature.

The last summary is a summary allowing you to visualize the receipts and to see those which make you want.

Symbology:

The symbology is simple, each symbol has its meaning:

Kitchen tool :

Sometimes a recipe can be made by several different kitchen utensils. You choose !

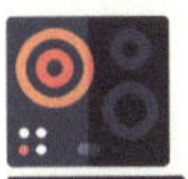 Using a hotplate

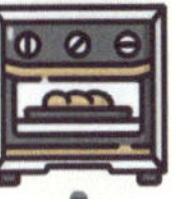 Use of the oven

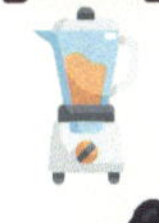 Using the blender

 Using the Mortar/Pestle

Use of the BBQ

Method of preparation:

In general, for 100g:

In a mortar, pour 90 grams of good quality salt *(coarse salt)* and 10 grams of spice or herb.

Grind the whole with a pestle to obtain a homogeneous mixture.

Then pour everything into a small jar to store it and treat your guests.

Conservation :

For salt and spice mixtures, the preservation is several months or even years depending on the spices, provided that the salt is kept away from light and humidity.

For salt and fruit/vegetable mixtures, the conservation is 2 to 4 months provided that the salt is stored away from light and humidity.

Summary by nomenclature

Thematic summary

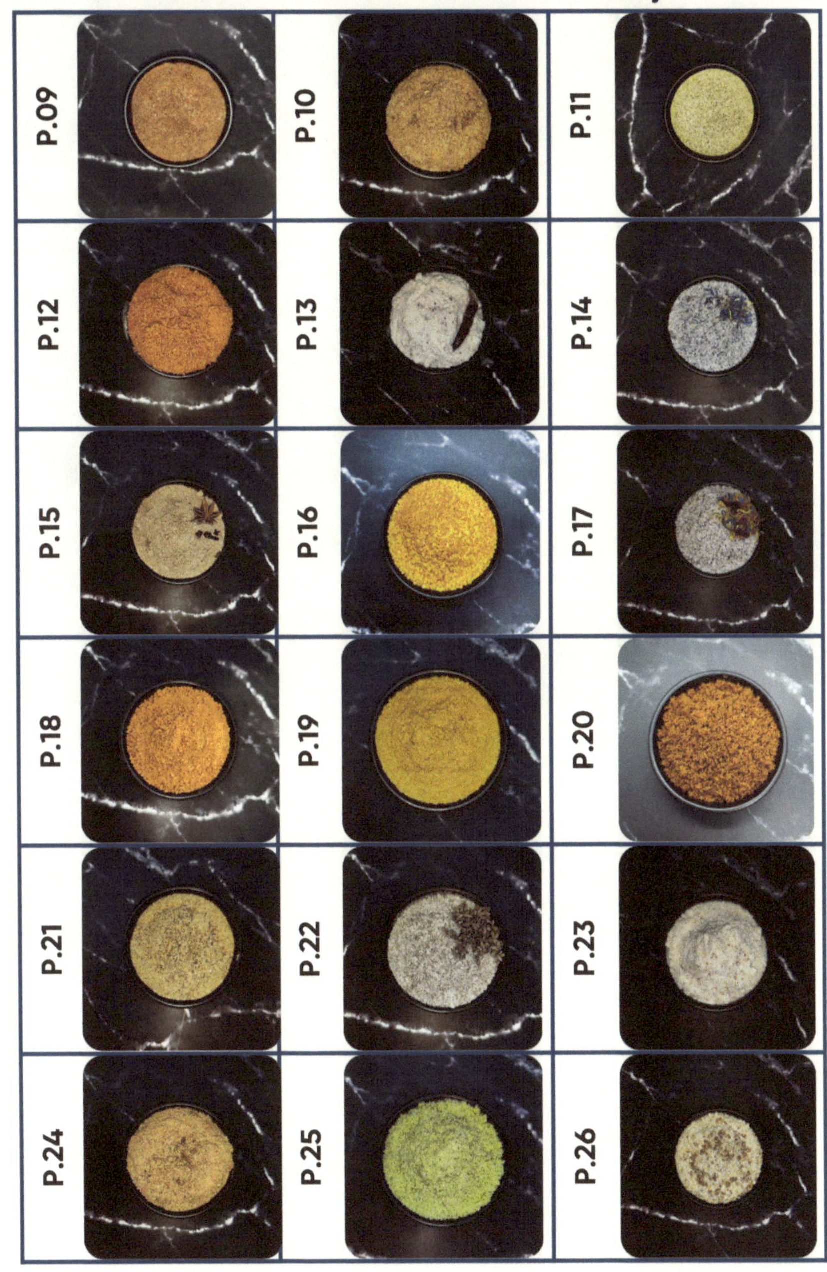

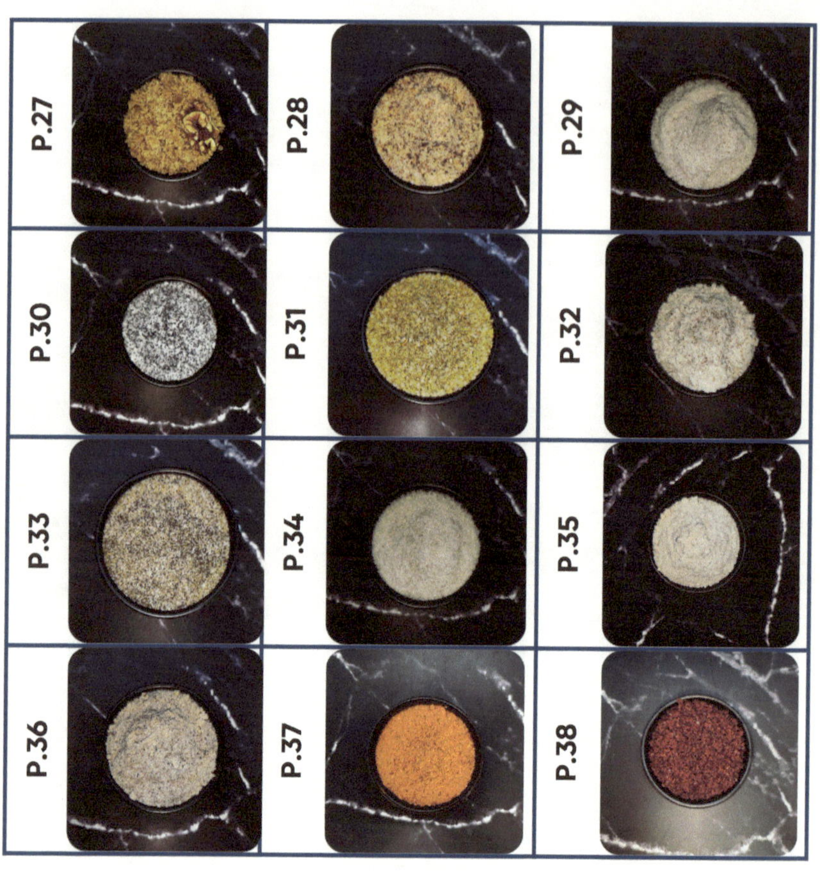

P.27
P.28
P.29
P.30
P.31
P.32
P.33
P.34
P.35
P.36
P.37
P.38

BBQ

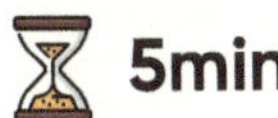

⏳ 5min

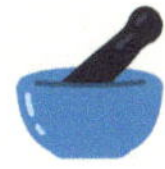

<u>Ingrédients :</u>
- 4 tablespoons smoked paprika
- 1 tablespoon of curry
- 1 teaspoon of hot pepper
- 1 teaspoon of coriander
- 1 teaspoon of pepper
- 1 teaspoon of thyme
- 2 teaspoon of cumin
- 70g of salt

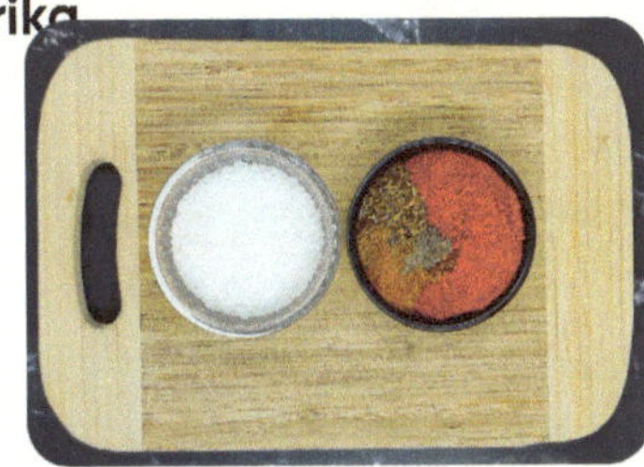

<u>Step 1 :</u>
- Mix everything

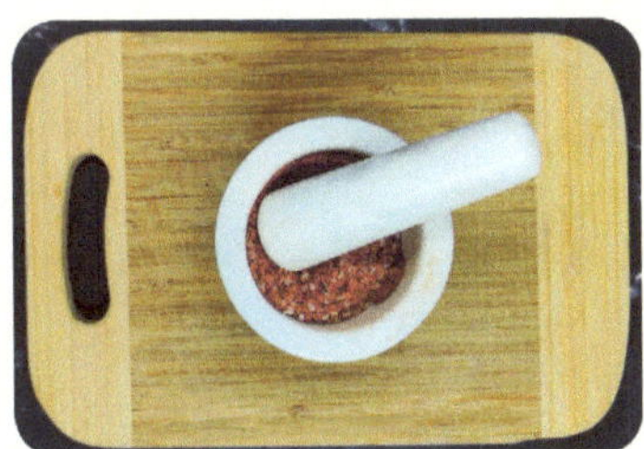

<u>Step 2 :</u>
- Crush everything with the mortar

<u>Step 3 :</u>
- Place in an airtight container.

<u>Ideal with:</u> meat and fish

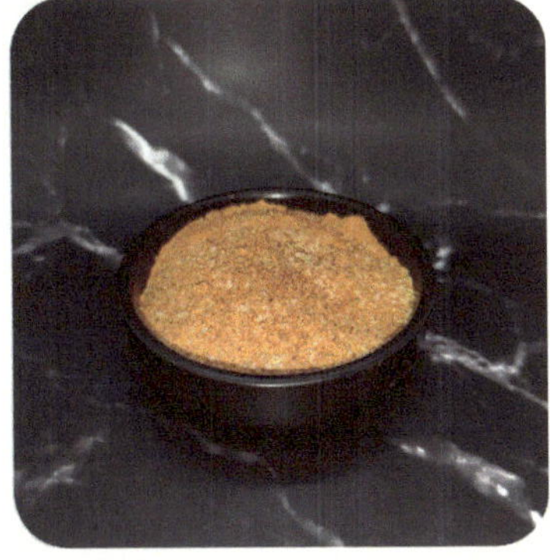

Caribbean

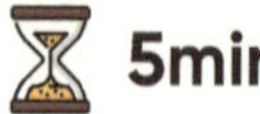 5min

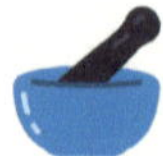

Ingrédients :
- 80g coarse salt
- 1 tablespoon chilli
- 1 tablespoon onion powder
- 1 teaspoon of turmeric
- 1 teaspoon of paprika
- 1 teaspoon of garlic

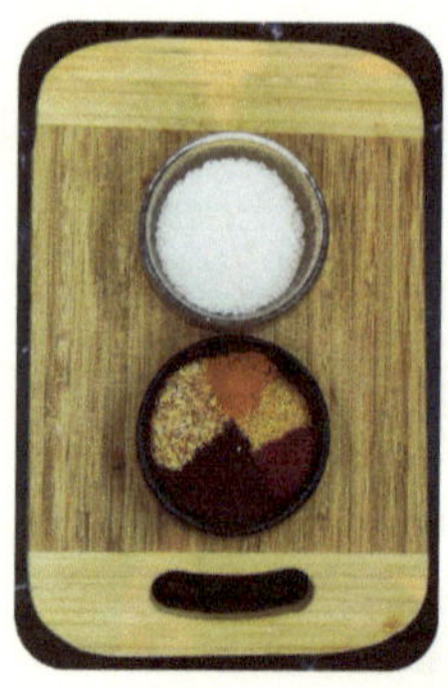

Step 1 :
- Mix everything

Step 2 :
- Crush everything with the mortar

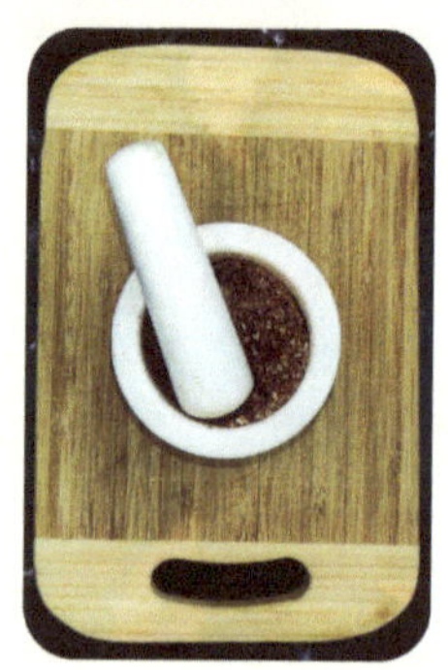

Step 3 :
- Put in an airtight container

Ideal with: meat and fish

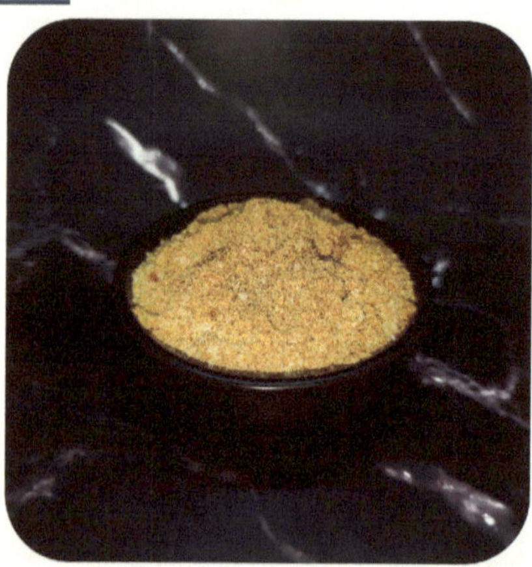

Celery

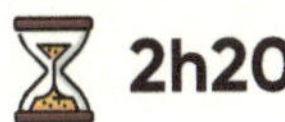

⏳ 2h20

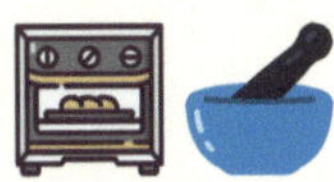

Ingrédients :
- 50g coarse salt
- 150g fresh celery

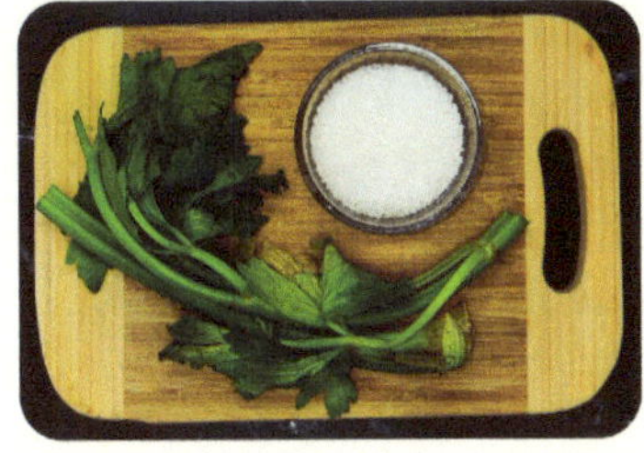

Step 1 :
- Preheat the oven to 90°C
- Finely chop the celery

Step 2 :
- Put on a baking sheet
- Put in the oven for 2 hours

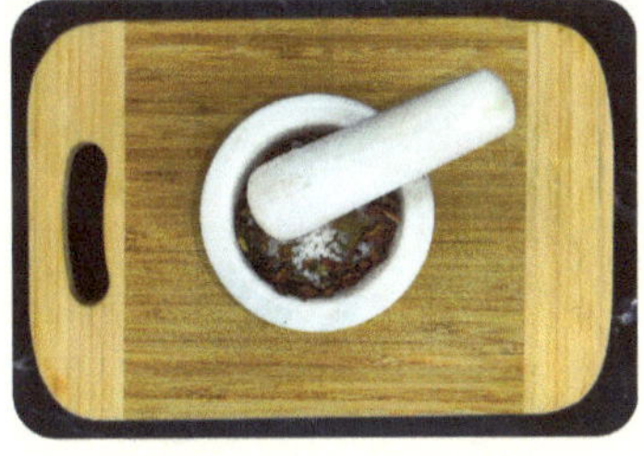

Step 3 :
- Mix the celery very finely

Step 4 :
- Crush everything with the mortar

Step 5 :
- Put in an airtight container

Ideal with: vegetable juice, salad, raw vegetables and cooked vegetables

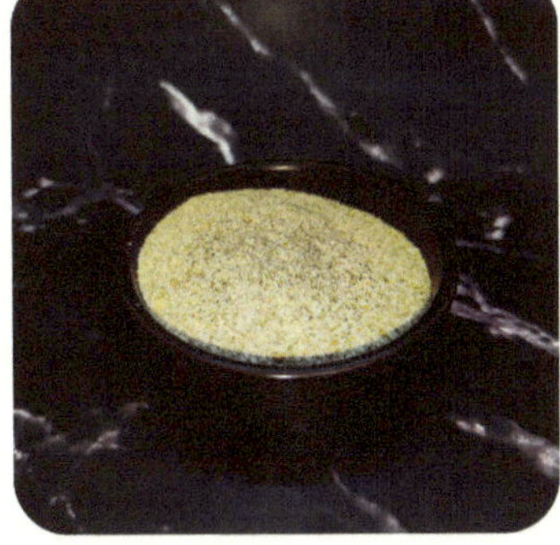

Chicken

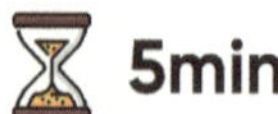

⏳ 5min

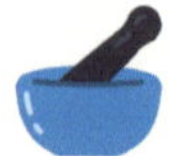

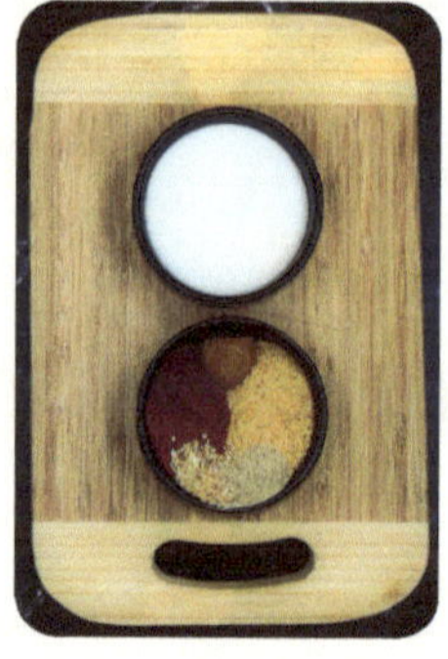

<u>Ingrédients :</u>
- 6 tablespoons fine salt
- 2 chicken stock cubes
- 3 tablespoons sweet paprika
- 3 tablespoon of garlic
- 1 teaspoon of white pepper
- 1 tablespoon onion powder

<u>Step 1 :</u>
- Mix everything

<u>Step 2 :</u>
- Crush everything with the mortar

<u>Step 3 :</u>
- Put in an airtight container

<u>Ideal with:</u> fries, potatoes and chicken

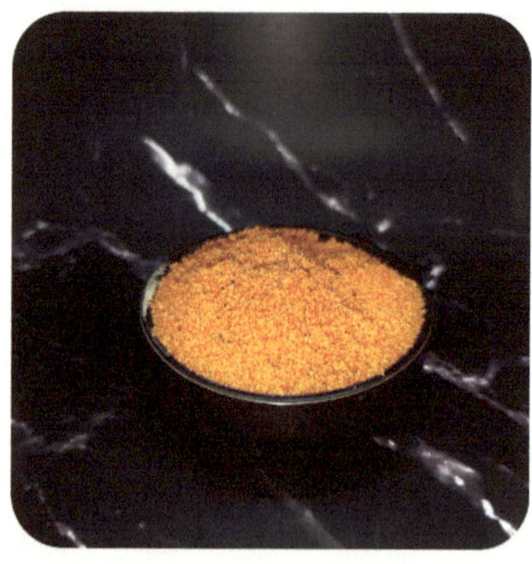

Chilli pepper

 2h50

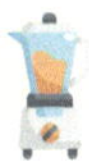

<u>Ingrédients :</u>
- 3 red cayenne peppers
- 100g salt

<u>Step 1 :</u>
- Mix the salt and pepper

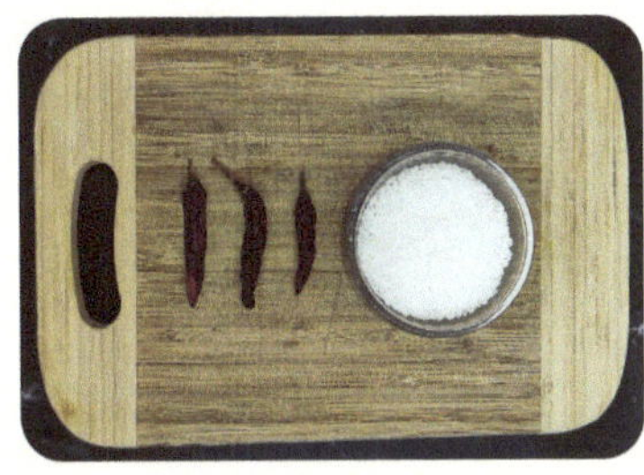

<u>Step 2 :</u>
- Mix everything

⚠️ <u>Warning</u> ⚠️ : open the blender after 10 minutes and preferably outdoors. Chilli micro-powder can be volatile and obstruct the airways for a short time.
Once these particles are gone, there is no more danger

<u>Step 3 :</u>
- Put in an airtight container

<u>Ideal with:</u> all types of dishes

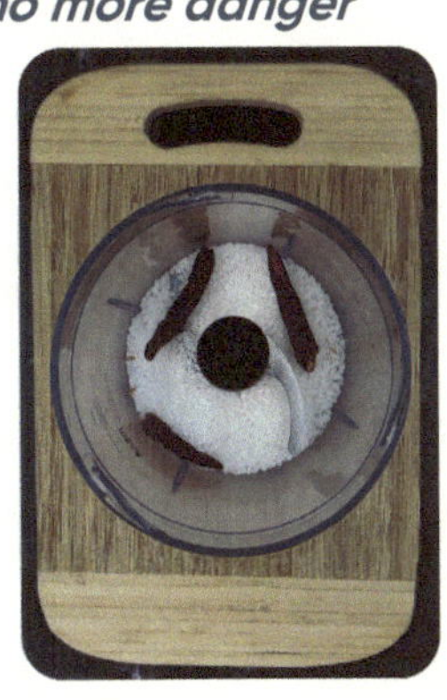

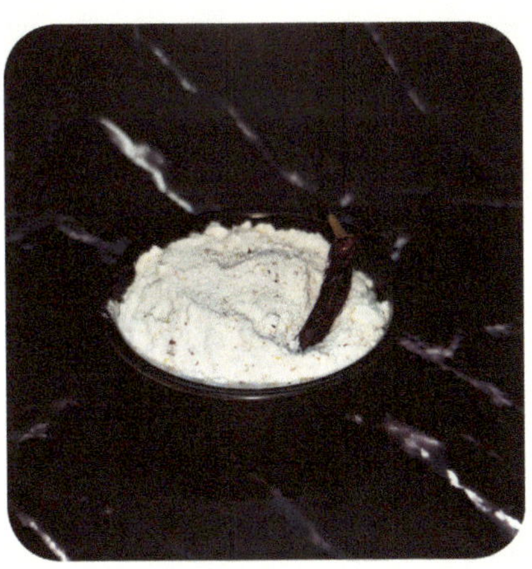

Cornflower

 5min

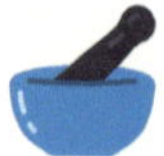

Ingrédients :
- 50g salt
- 1 handful of dried cornflowers

Step 1 :
- Mix everything

Step 2 :
- Crush everything with the mortar

Step 3 :
- Put in an airtight container

Ideal with: fish and chicken

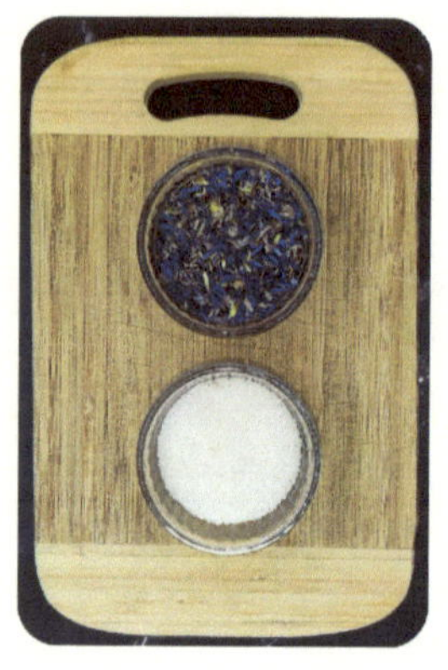

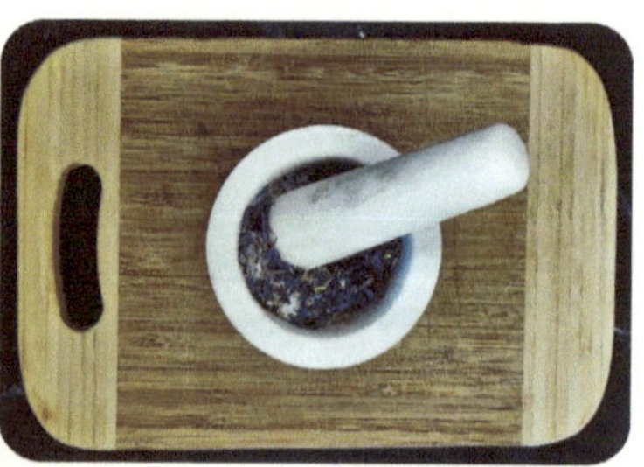

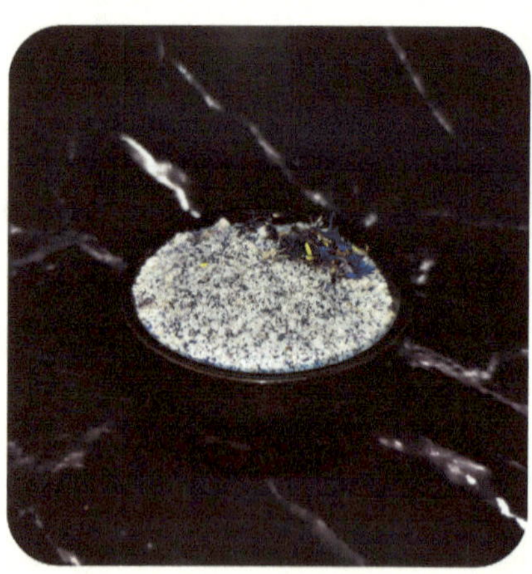

Christmas salt

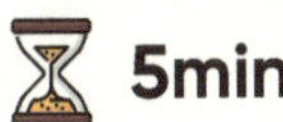 5min

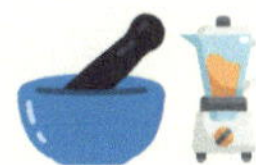

Ingrédients :
- 2 teaspoon of cinnamon
- ½ teaspoon of ginger
- 6 cloves
- 2 cardamom pods
- ½ star anise
- 70g coarse salt

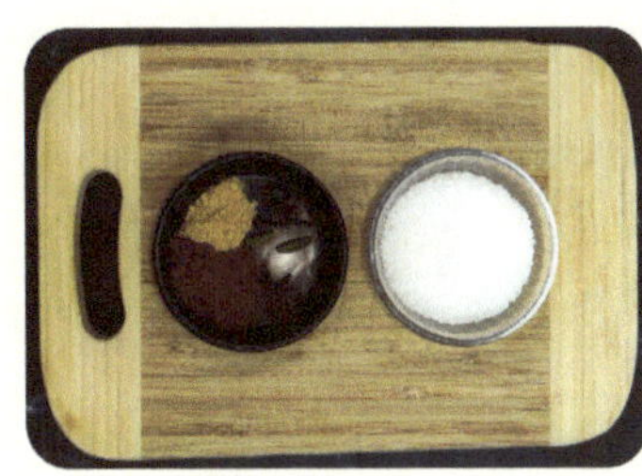

Step 1 :
- Shell the cardamom seeds to keep only the black seeds
- Mix all the spices

Step 2 :
- Mix spices and salt

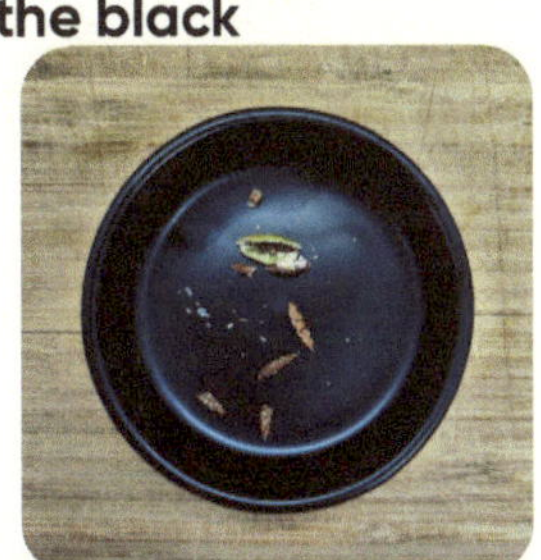

Step 3 :
- Crush with the mortar

Step 4 :
- Put in an airtight container

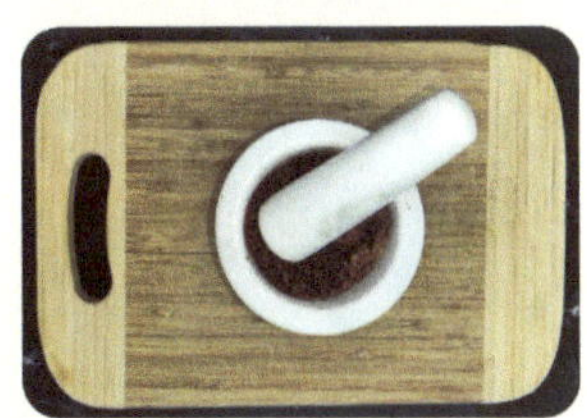

Ideal with: white meat

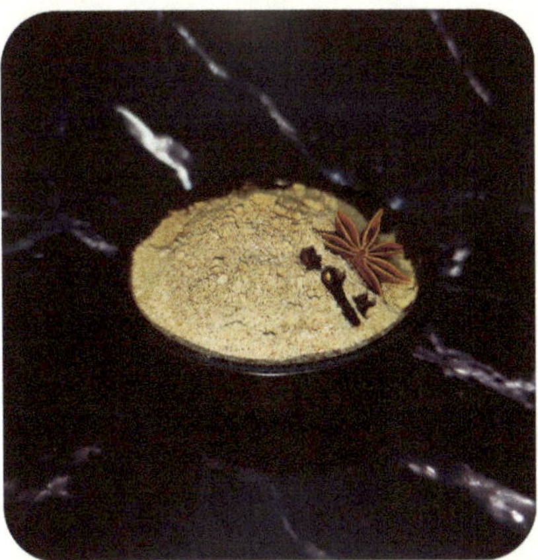

Curry

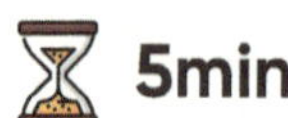
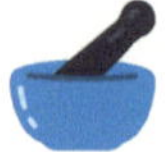

Ingrédients :
- 90g coarse salt
- 10g of curry

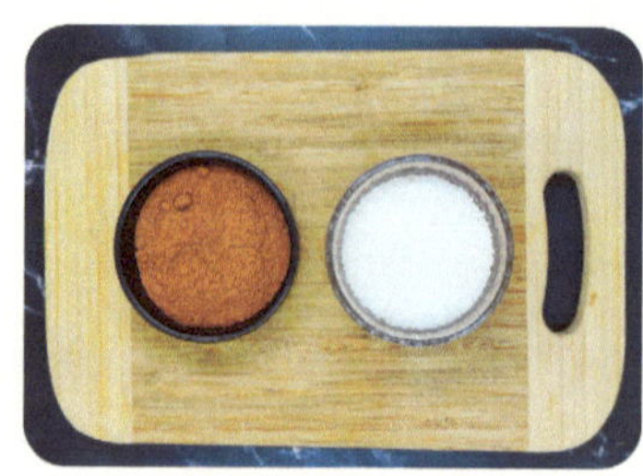

Step 1 :
- Mix everything

Step 2 :
- Crush everything with the mortar

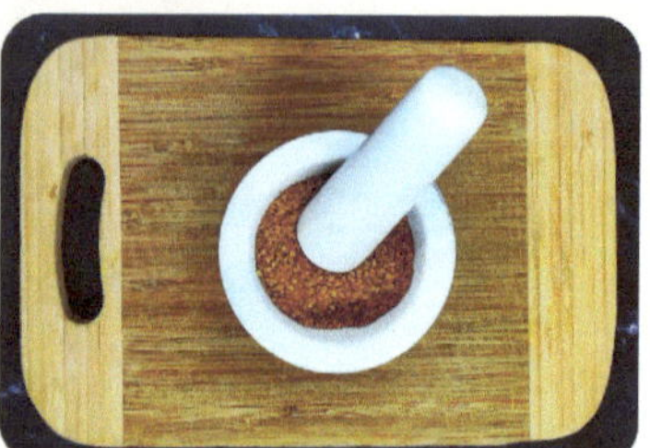

Step 3 :
- Put in an airtight container

Ideal with: fries, potatoes, fish and white meat

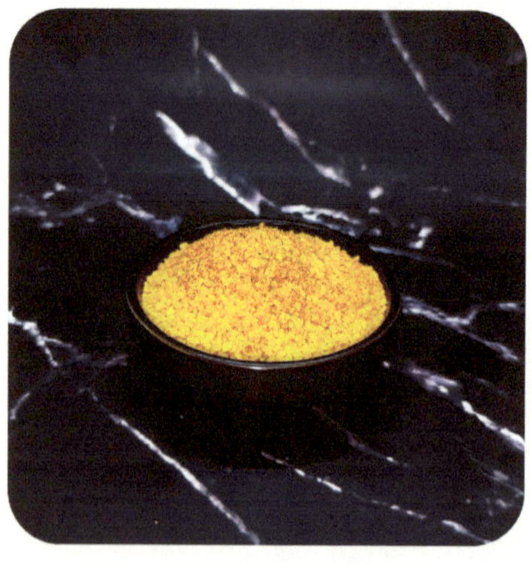

Flowery

 5min

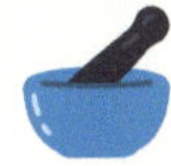

Ingrédients :
- 1 handful of dried edible flower mix
- 80g coarse salt

Step 1 :
- Mix everything

Step 2 :
- Crush everything with the mortar

Step 3 :
- Put in an airtight container

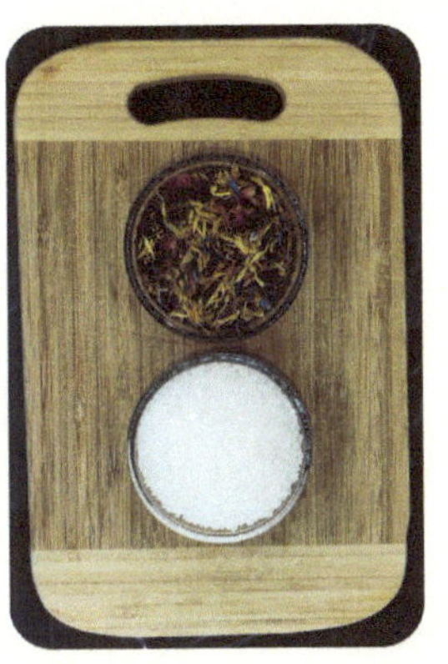

Ideal with: fish and raw vegetables

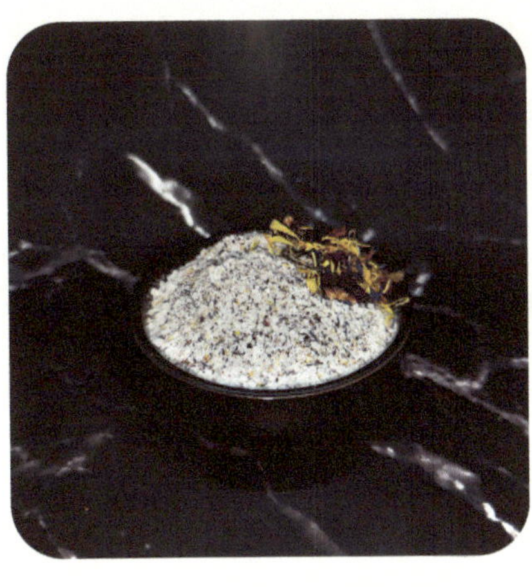

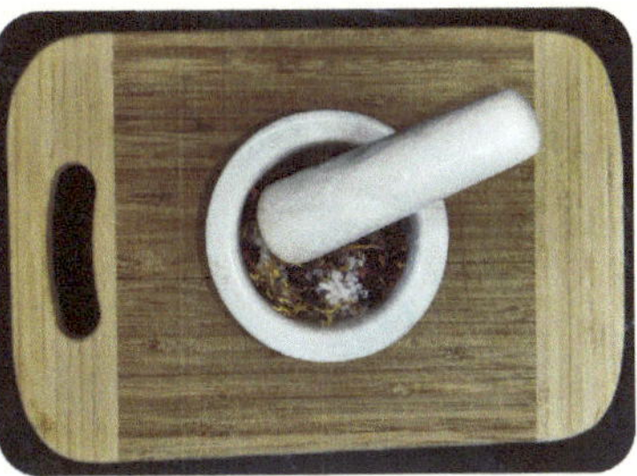

Garlic

 4h

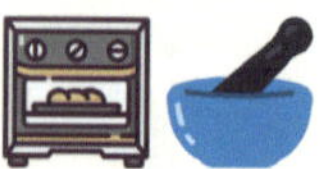

Ingrédients :
- 1 garlic
- 150g coarse salt
- Olive oil

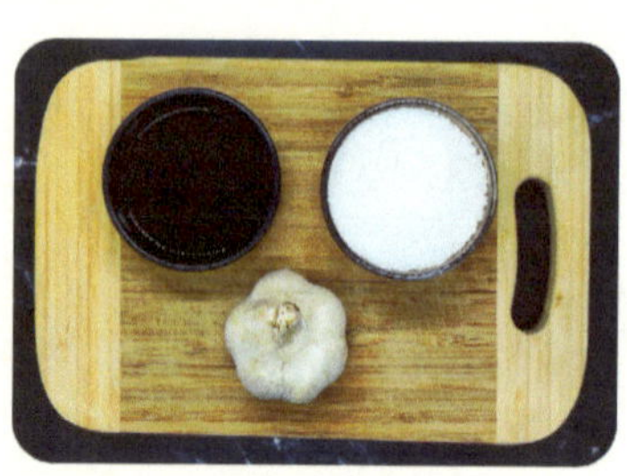

Step 1 :
- Preheat the oven to 180°C
- Cut the head of the garlic
- Enclose the garlic in aluminum with a little olive oil
- Put the garlic in the oven for 1 hour

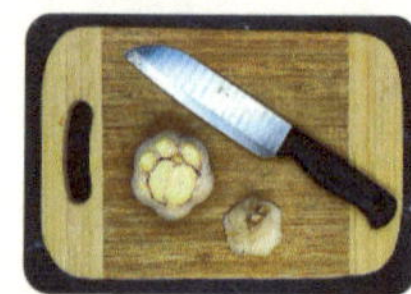

Step 2 :
- Degerminate/empty the garlic
- Mix the garlic purée and the salt

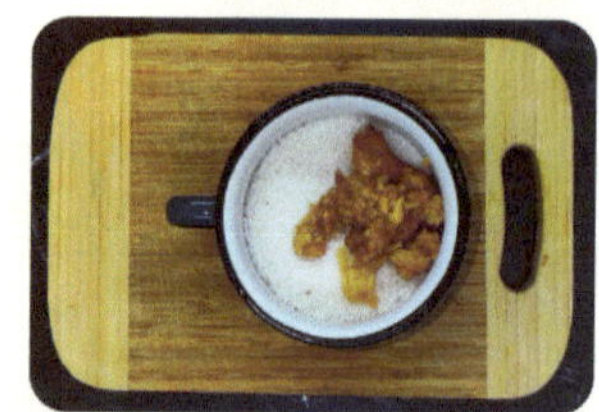

Step 3 :
- Preheat the oven to 90°C
- Spread the mixture on a baking sheet
- Put in the oven for 2h30
The dough will become dry and hard

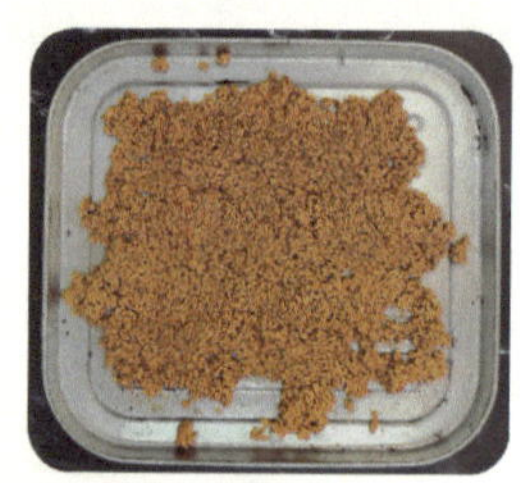

Step 4 :
- Break the dough into small pieces
- Finish the job with the mortar

Step 5 :
- Store in an airtight container

Ideal with: white meat, fish and vegetables

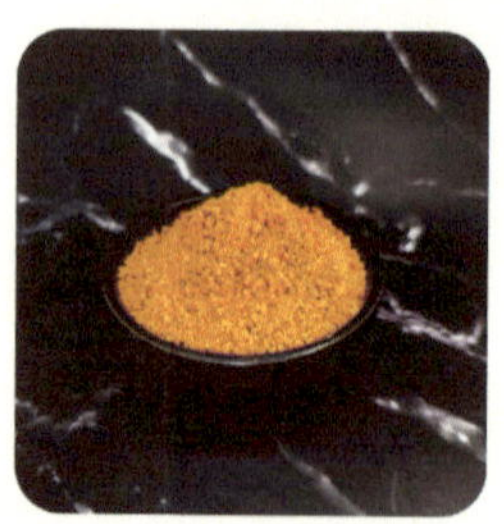

Ginger

⏳ 5min

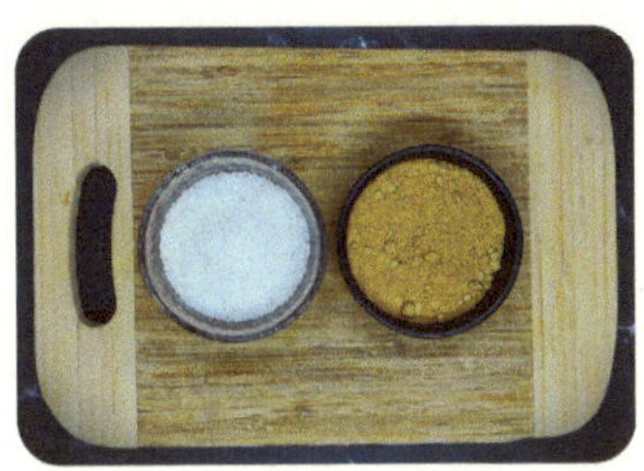

Ingrédients :
- 10g powdered ginger
- 90g coarse salt

Step 1 :
- Mix everything

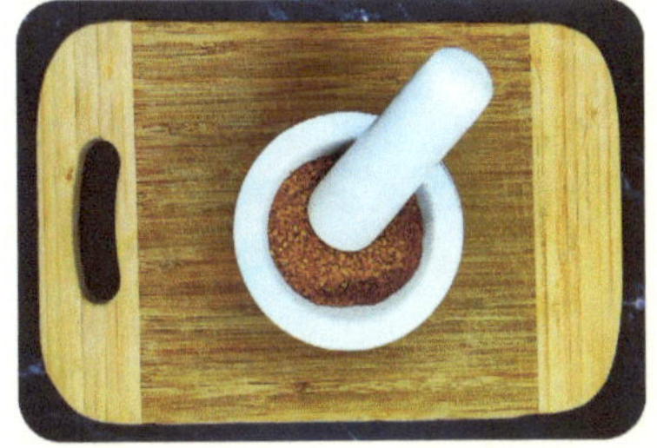

Step 2 :
- Crush everything with the mortar

Step 3 :
- Put in an airtight container

Ideal with: fish, chicken, shellfish and fruit

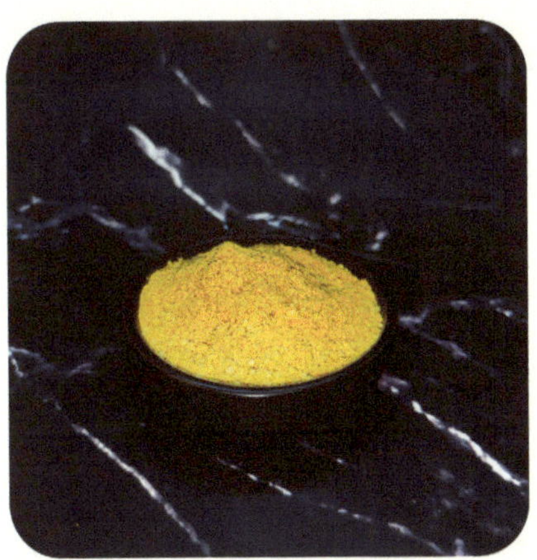

Gomasio

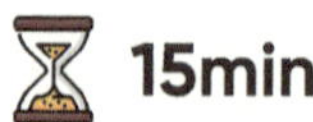 15min

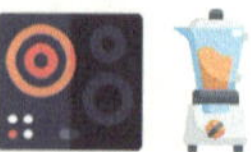

<u>Ingrédients :</u>
- 10g coarse salt
- 90g sesame seeds

<u>Step 1 :</u>
- Mix everything
- Grill everything in a pan for 5 minutes

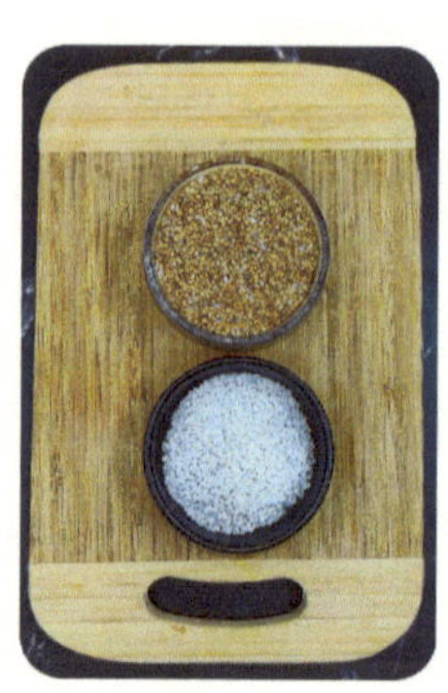

<u>Step 2 :</u>
- Mix everything finely in stages

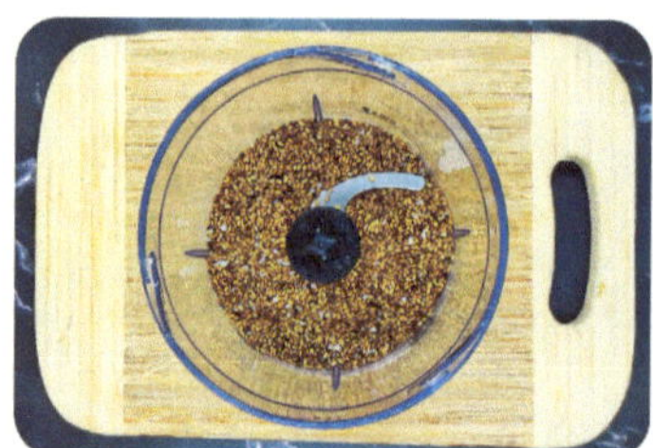

<u>Step 3 :</u>
- Put in an airtight container

<u>Ideal with:</u> vinaigrette, raw vegetables, meat, fish, vegetables, salad, bread, soup and cereal

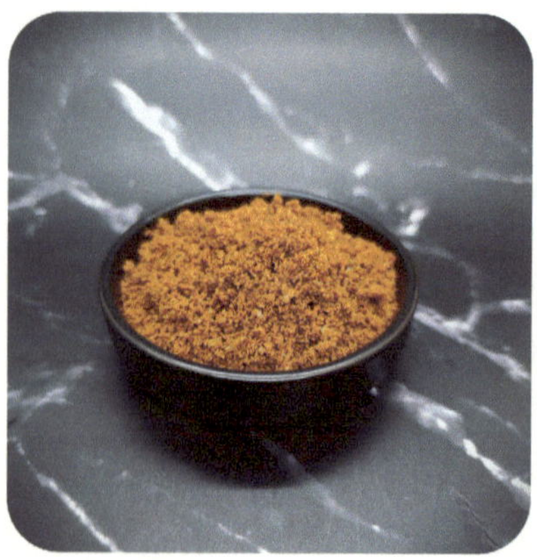

Kumquat

 3h20

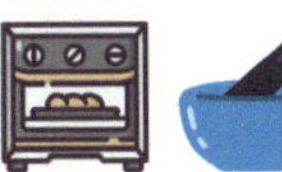

Ingrédients :
- 5 – 10 Kumquats
- 70g coarse salt

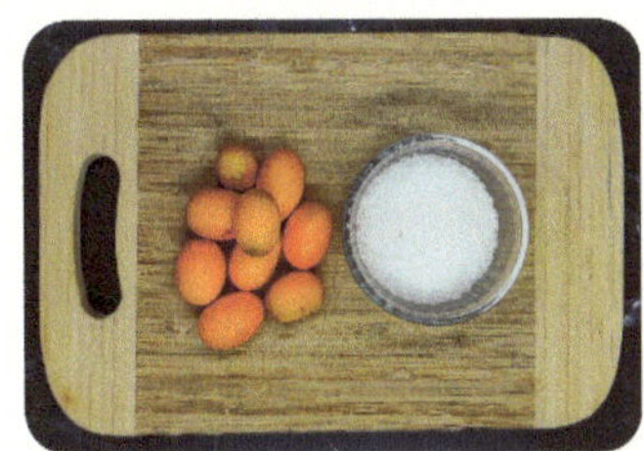

Step 1 :
- Preheat the oven to 90°
- Finely cut the kumquats

Step 2 :
- Étaler les morceaux sur une plaque de four
- Mettre au four pendant 3h

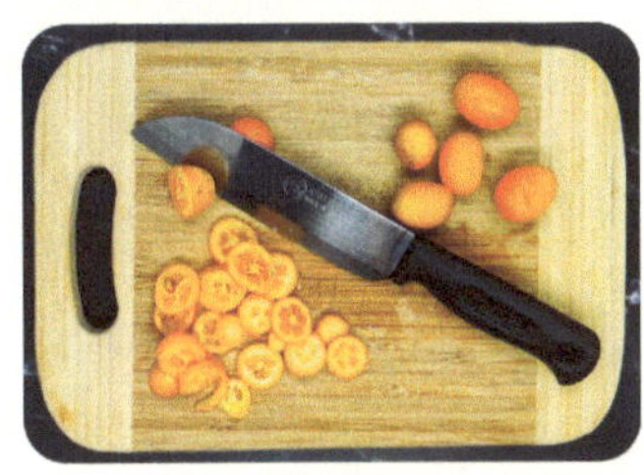

Step 3 :
- Lightly mix the kumquat pieces
- Mix the salt and the kumquats

Step 4 :
- Crush everything with the mortar

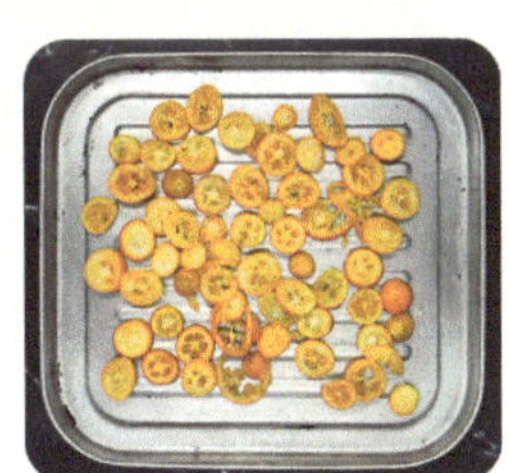

Step 5 :
- Put in an airtight container

Ideal with: fish and white meat

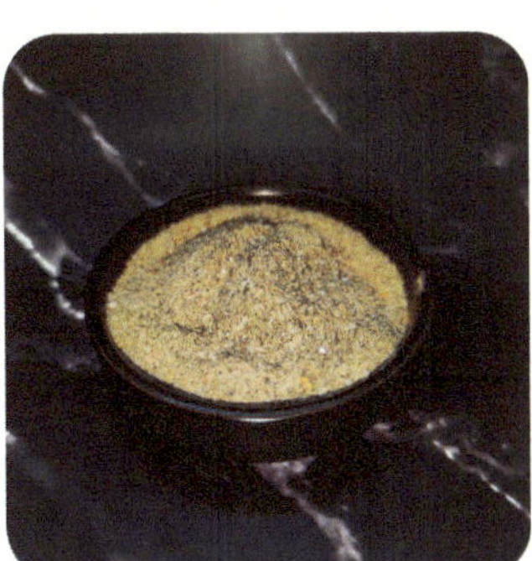

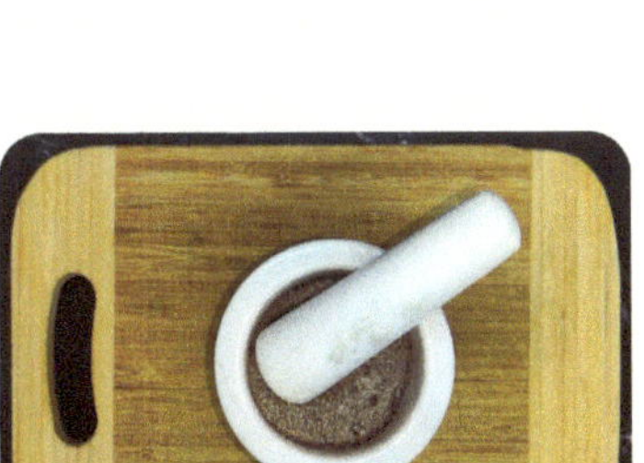

Lavender flower

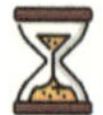 5min

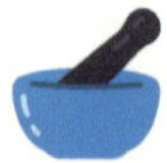

<u>Ingrédients :</u>
- 90g coarse salt
- 10g of dried lavender flower

<u>Step 1 :</u>
- Mix everything

<u>Step 2 :</u>
- Crush everything with the mortar

<u>Step 3 :</u>
- Place in an airtight container.

<u>Ideal with:</u> fish, pork and chicken

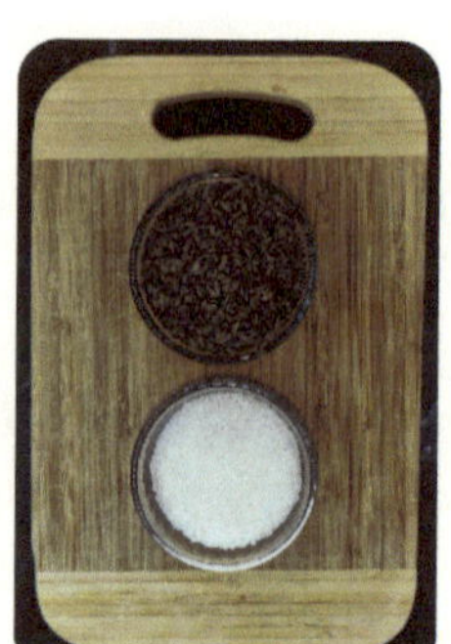

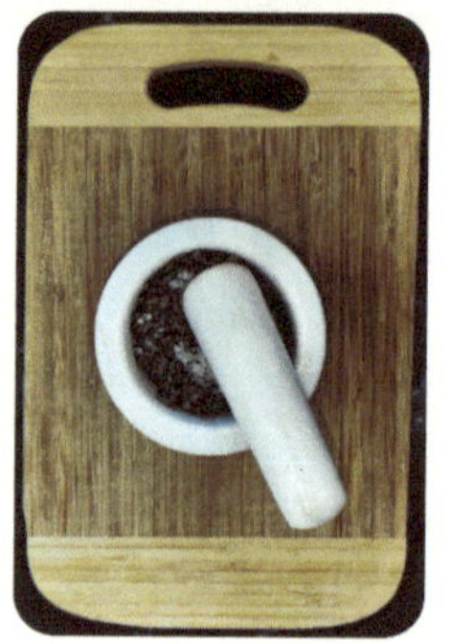

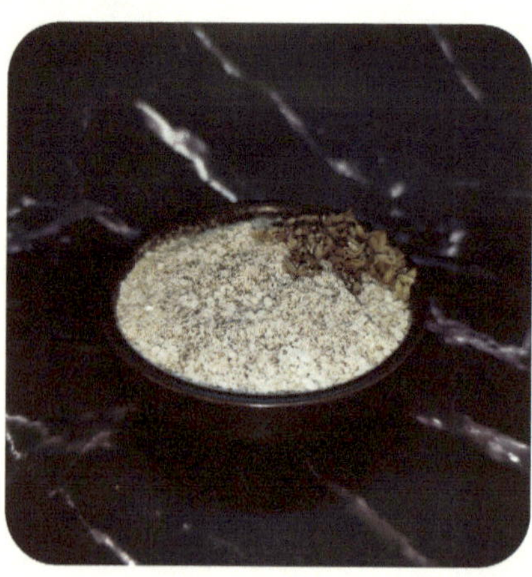

Lemon

 1h20

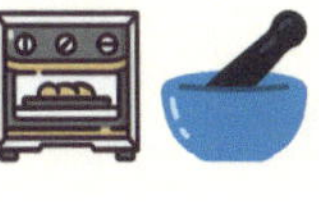

Ingrédients :
- 1 lemon
- 95g coarse salt

Step 1 :
- Preheat the oven to 90°
- Grate the lemon to make lemon zest

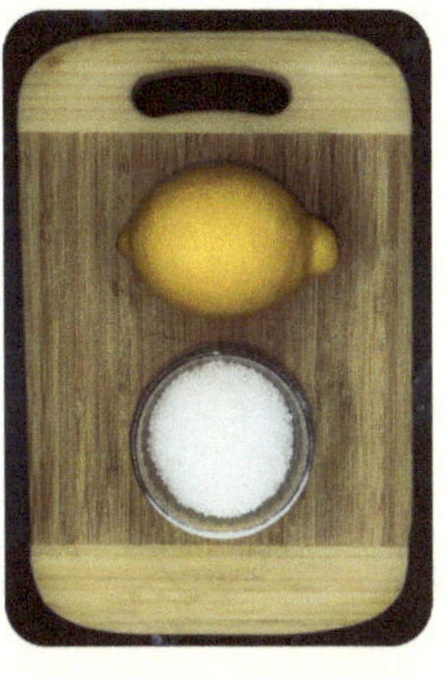

Step 2 :
- Spread the zest on a baking sheet
- Put in the oven for 1 hour

Step 3 :
- Mix the salt and lemon zest

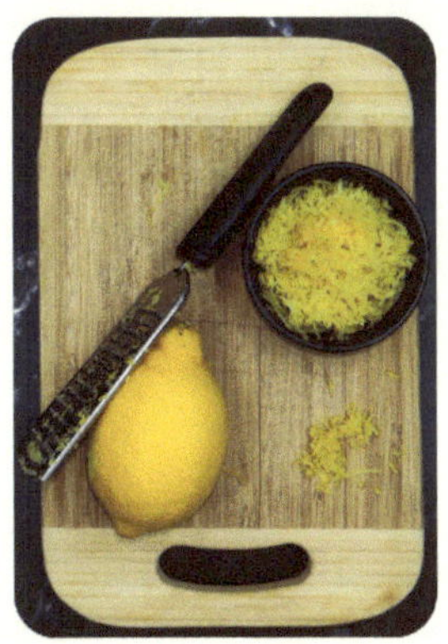

Step 4 :
- Crush everything with the mortar

Step 5 :
- Put in an airtight container

Ideal with: fish and rice

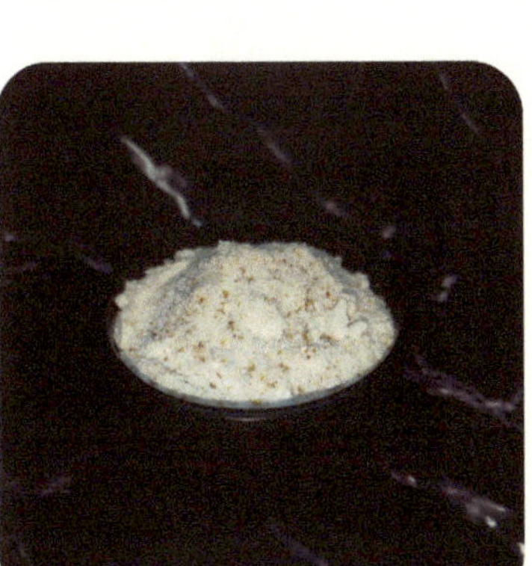

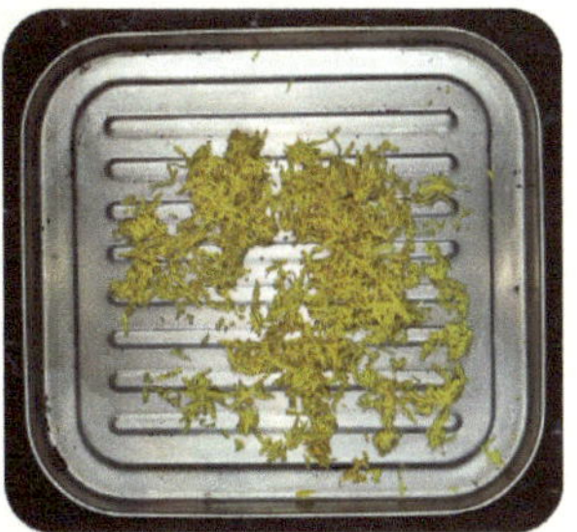

Meat

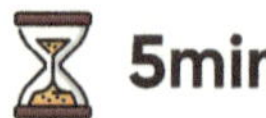 5min

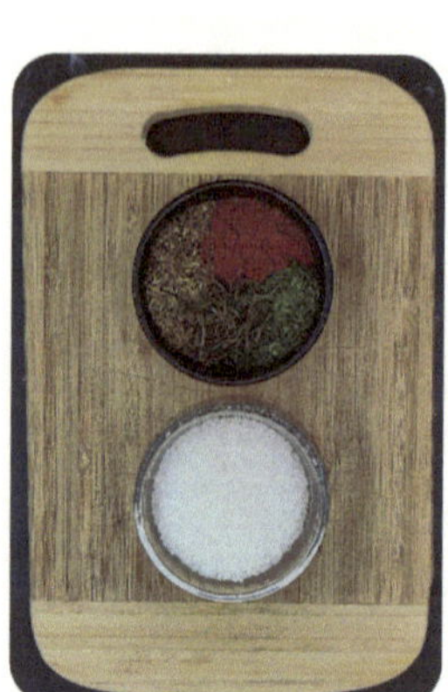

<u>Ingrédients :</u>
- 1 tablespoon of 5 berries
- 2 teaspoon sweet paprika
- 1 teaspoon of thyme
- 1 teaspoon of coriander
- 1 teaspoon of dried rosemary
- 90g coarse salt

<u>Step 1 :</u>
- Mix all the ingredients

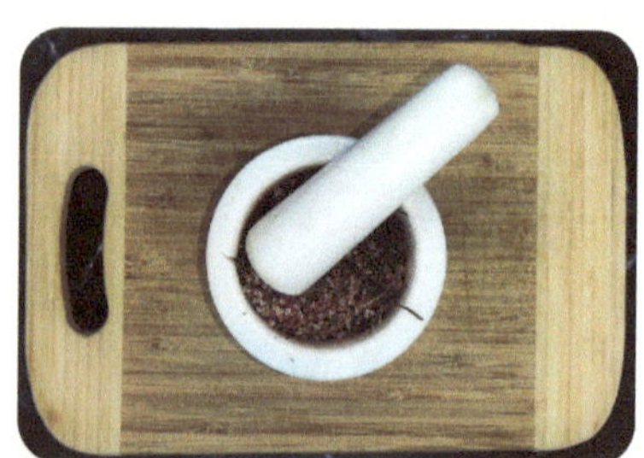

<u>Step 2 :</u>
- Crush everything in a mortar
- Put in an airtight container

<u>Ideal with:</u> red meat

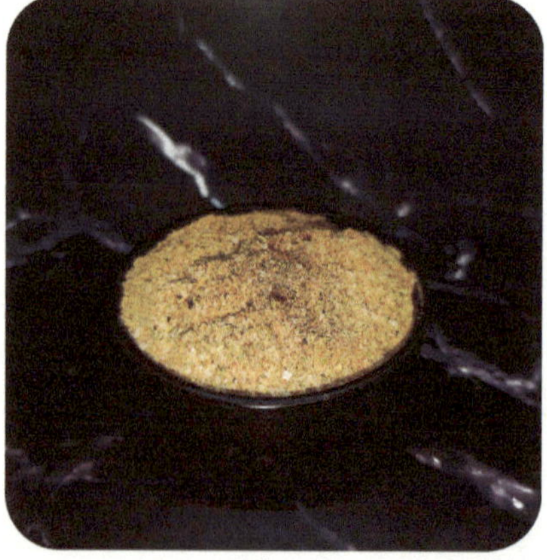

Menthol

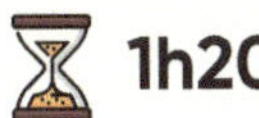

⏳ 1h20

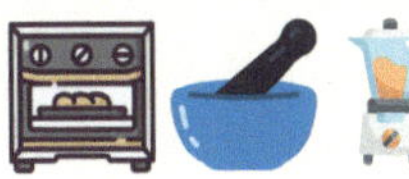

Ingrédients :
- **About fifteen mint leaves**
- **100g coarse salt**

Step 1 :
- **Preheat the oven to 90°**
- **Mix the salt and the mint**
- **Mix the salt and the mint leaves**
- **Put in the oven for 1 hour**

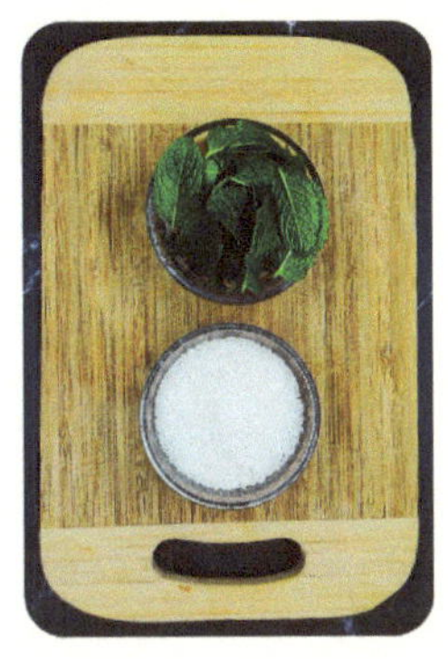

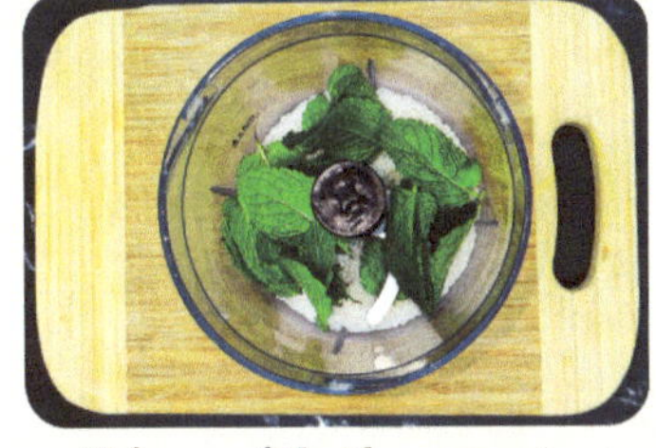

Step 2 :
- **Crush everything with the mortar**

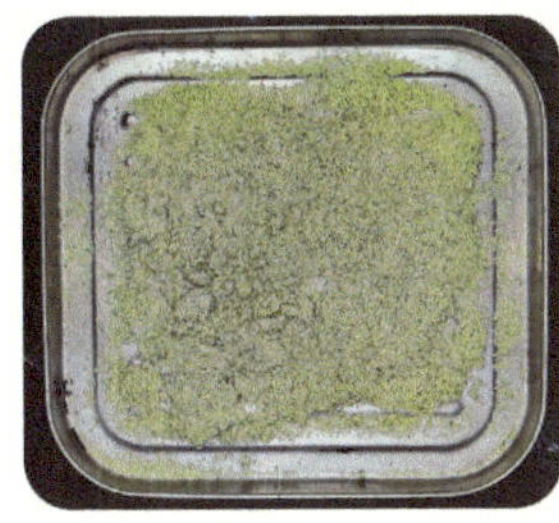

Step 3 :
- **Put in an airtight container**

Ideal with: **couscous, white meat and tabbouleh**

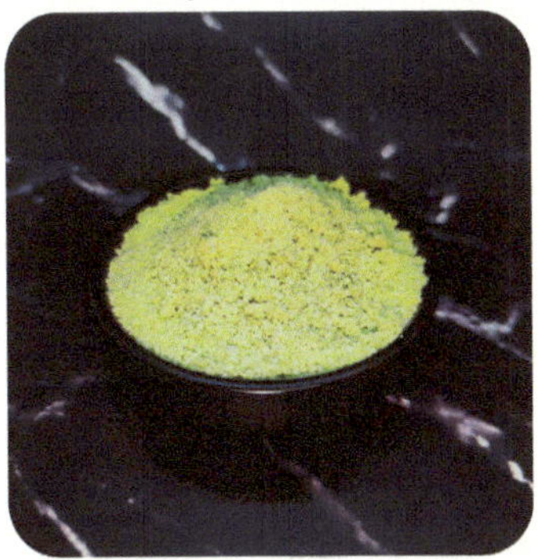

Mustard

 5min

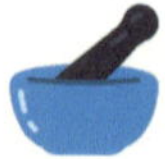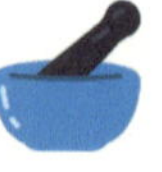

Ingrédients :
- 30g mustard seeds
- 70g salt

Step 1 :
- Mix everything

Step 2 :
- Crush everything with the mortar

Step 3 :
- Put in an airtight container

Ideal with: vegetables, raw vegetables, salad, meat and fish

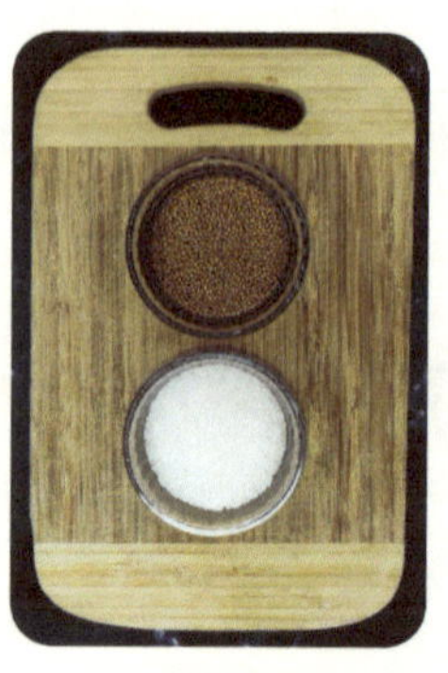

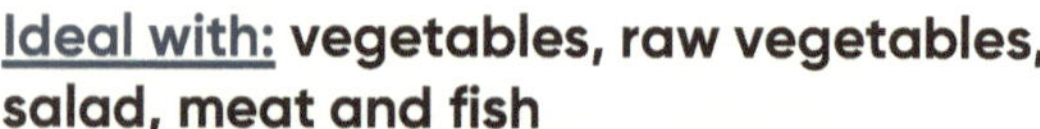

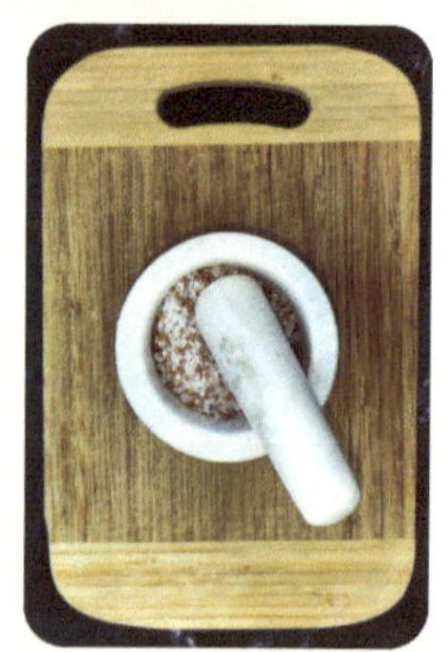

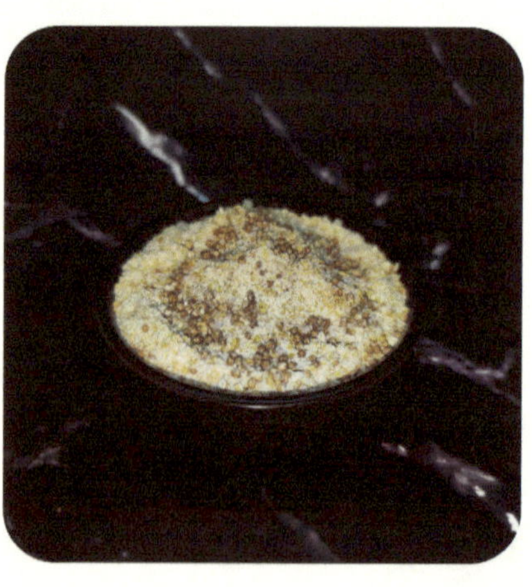

Nut

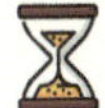 40min

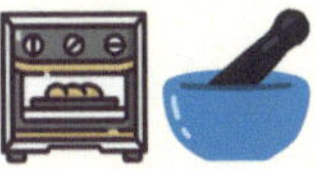

Ingrédients :
- 20g walnuts
- 80g coarse salt
- 1 teaspoon walnut oil

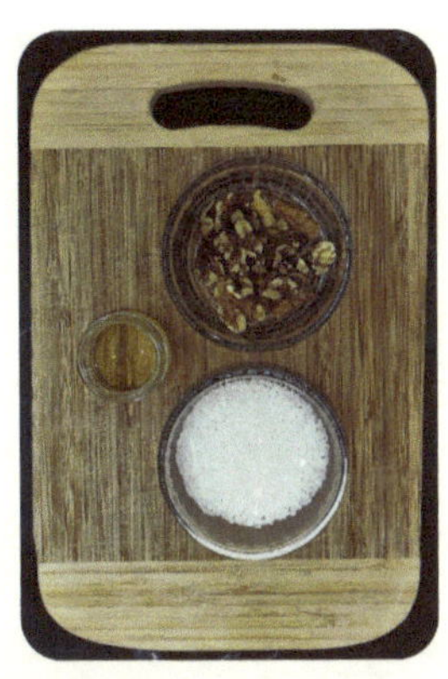

Step 3 :
- Preheat the oven to 90°C
- Mix everything
- Crush the mixture with the mortar

Step 3 :
- Spread on a baking sheet
- Put in the oven for 30min

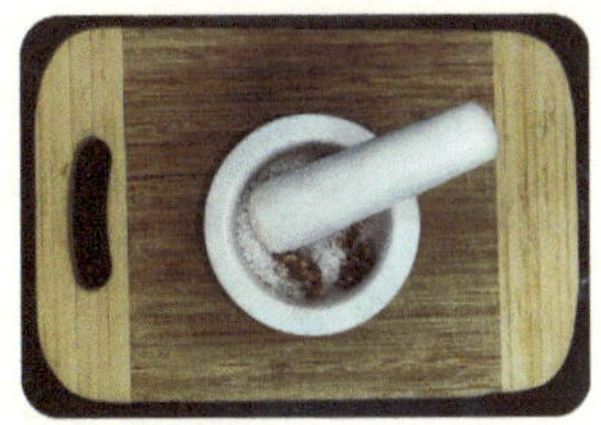

Step 3 :
- Put in an airtight container

Ideal with: mushrooms, raw vegetables, game and veal

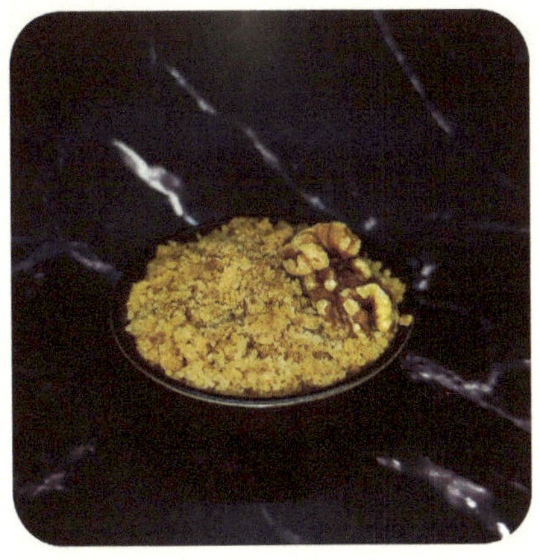

Pineapple

 3h30

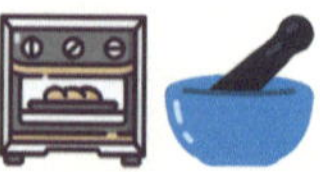

Ingrédients :
- 150g pineapple *(without skin)*
- 70g coarse salt

Step 1 :
- Preheat oven to 90°C
- Remove the pineapple skin
- Cut the pineapple into a thin slice

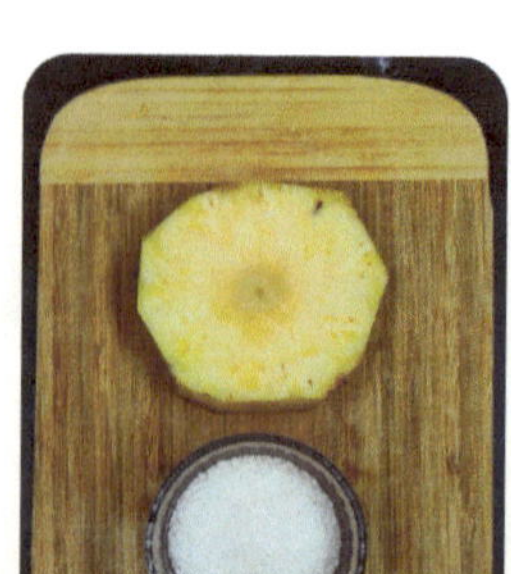

Step 2 :
- Put the slices on a baking sheet
- Flatten the slices with a fork
- Put in the oven for 2 hours
The pieces also caramelize

Step 3 :
- Break it into small pieces

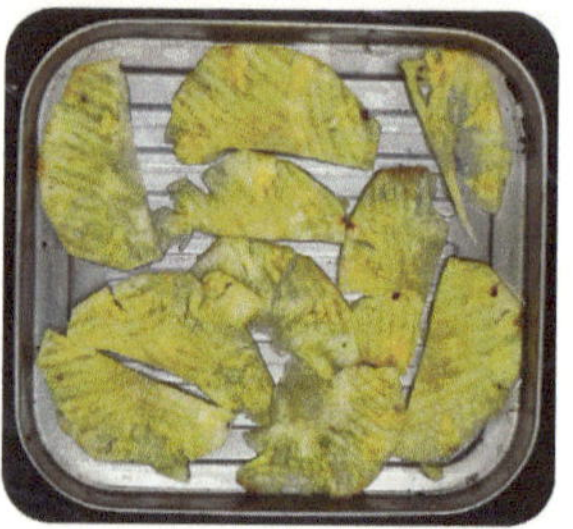

Step 4 :
- Mix the salt and the pineapple shavings
- Reduce everything with mortar

Step 5 :
- Put in an airtight container

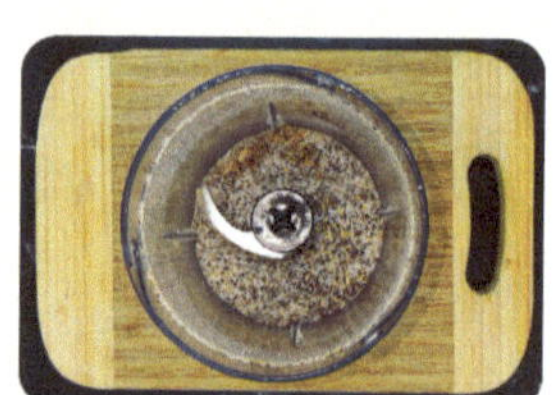

Ideal with: starter, dessert
and white meat

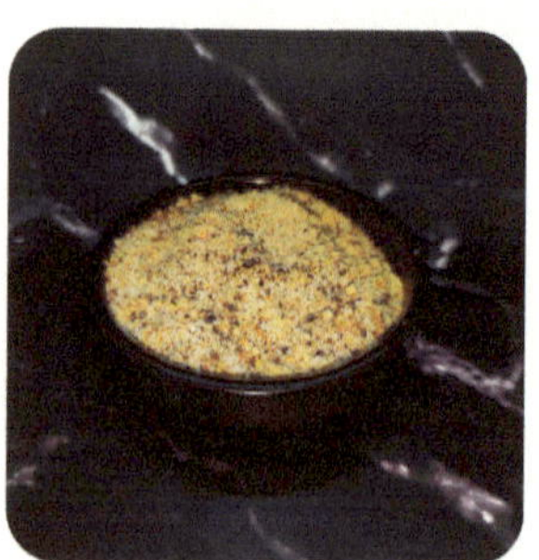

Pirate

 45min

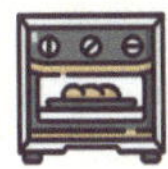

<u>Ingrédients :</u>
- 5cl old rum or spiced rum
- 100g salt

<u>Step 1 :</u>
- Preheat the oven to 90°C
- Mix it all together

<u>Step 2 :</u>
- Place on a baking tray
- Bake for 30 minutes

<u>Step 3 :</u>
- Place on a baking tray
- Bake for 30 minutes

<u>Ideal with:</u> fish, veal and pork

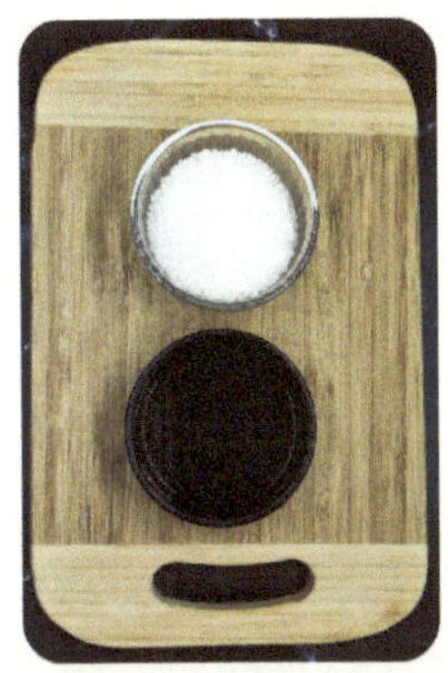

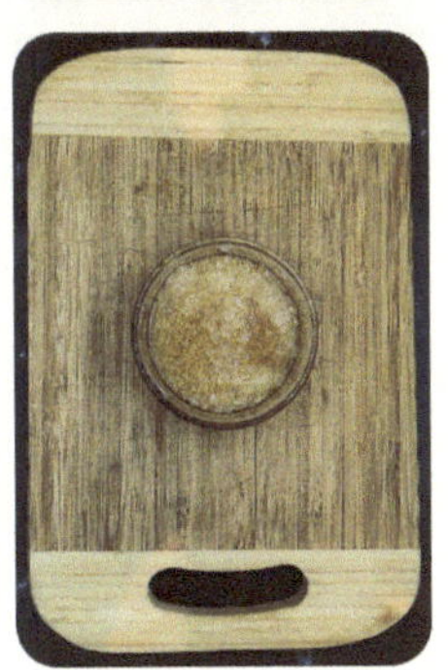

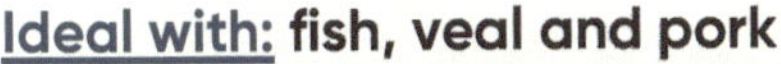

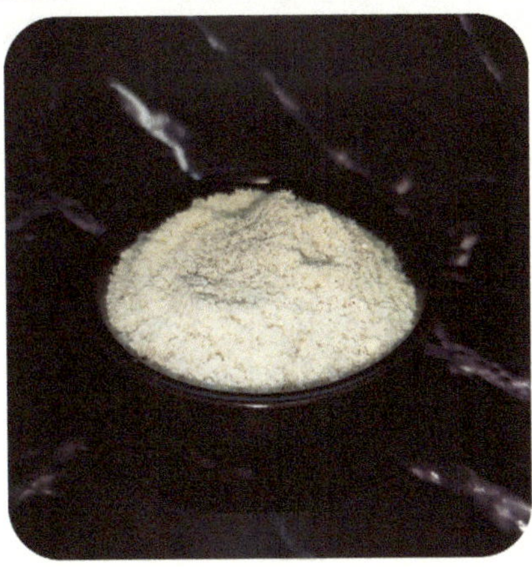

Poppy

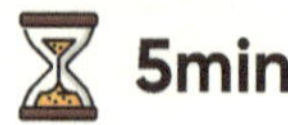 5min

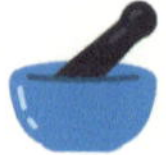

<u>Ingrédients :</u>
- 30g of poppy seeds
- 70g coarse salt

<u>Step 1 :</u>
- Mix everything

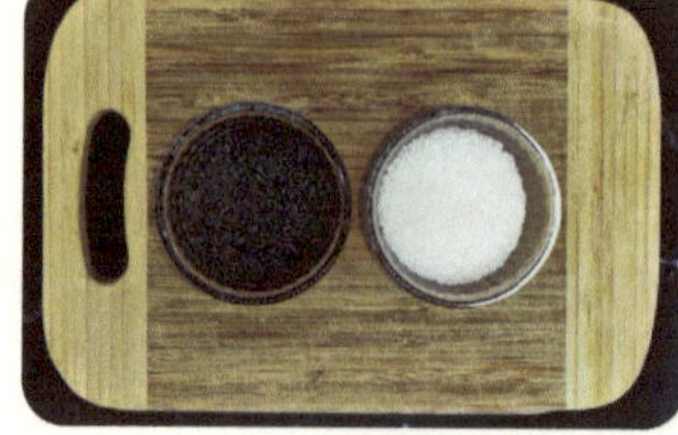

<u>Step 2 :</u>
- Grind the mix with the mortar

<u>Step 3 :</u>
- Put in an airtight container

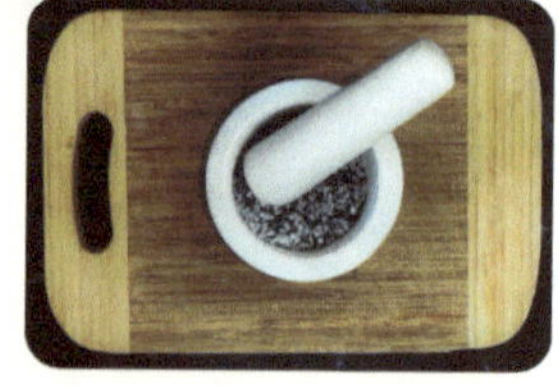

<u>Ideal with:</u> raw vegetables, salad, focaccia, brioche, pretzels and fish

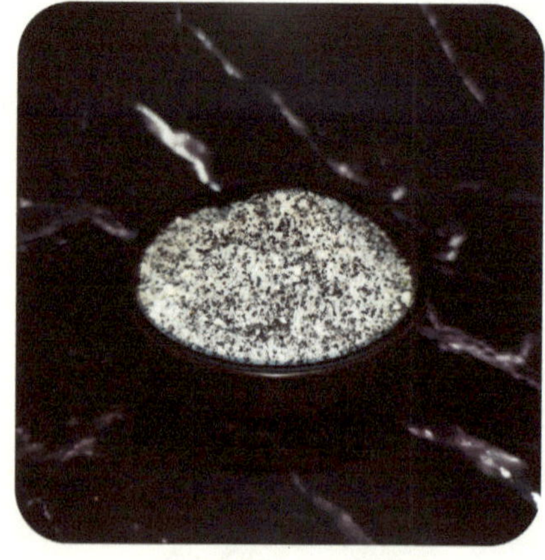

Provencal herbs

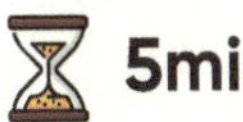 5min

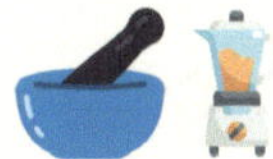

<u>Ingrédients :</u>
- 10g of Provencal herbs
- 90g coarse salt

<u>Step 1 :</u>
- Lightly mix the Provencal herbs
- Mix everything

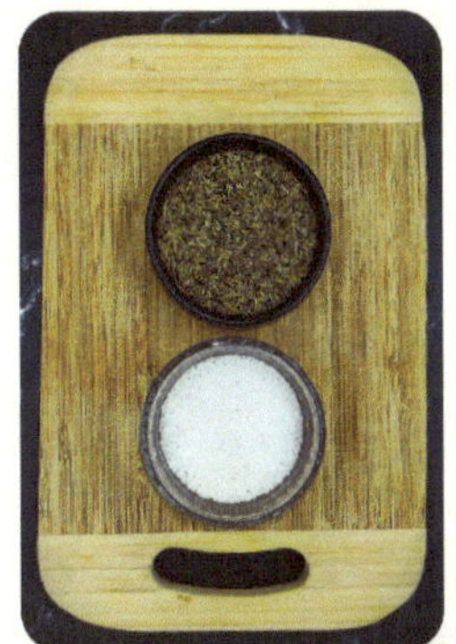

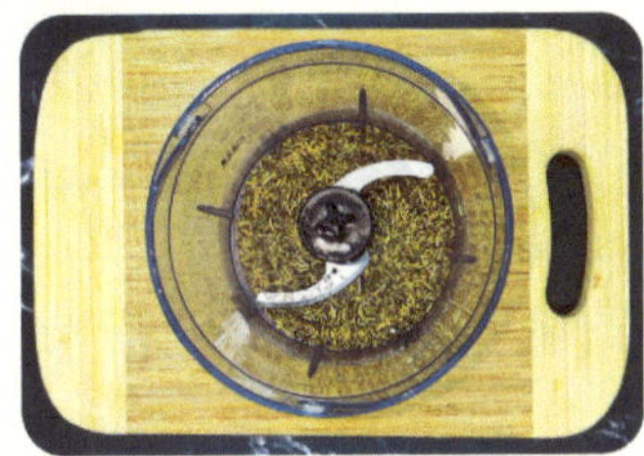

<u>Step 2 :</u>
- Crush everything with the mortar

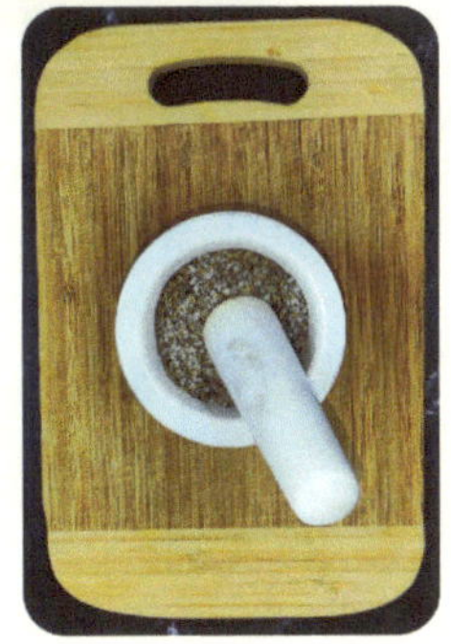

<u>Step 3 :</u>
- Put in an airtight container

<u>Ideal with:</u> vegetables, raw vegetables, meat and fish

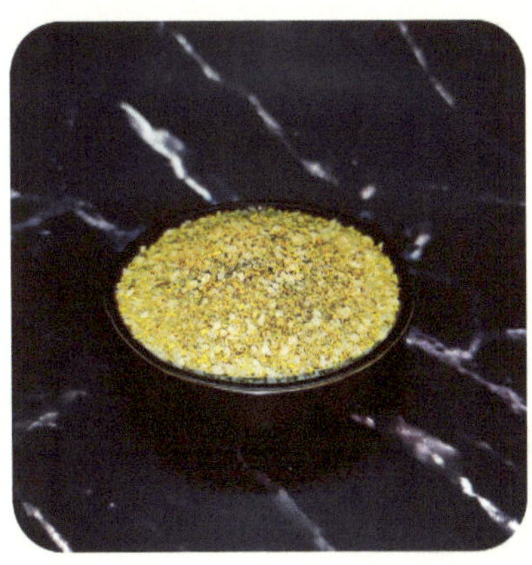

Rosemary Lemon

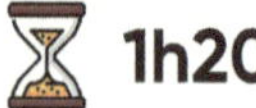 1h20

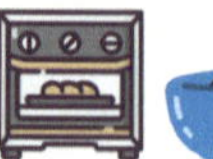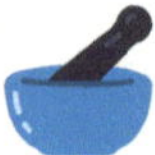

<u>Ingrédients :</u>
- 90gr coarse salt
- 4 teaspoons of fresh rosemary
- 1 lemon

<u>Step 1 :</u>
- Preheat the oven to 90°
- Grate the lemon to make lemon zest
- Finely chop the rosemary

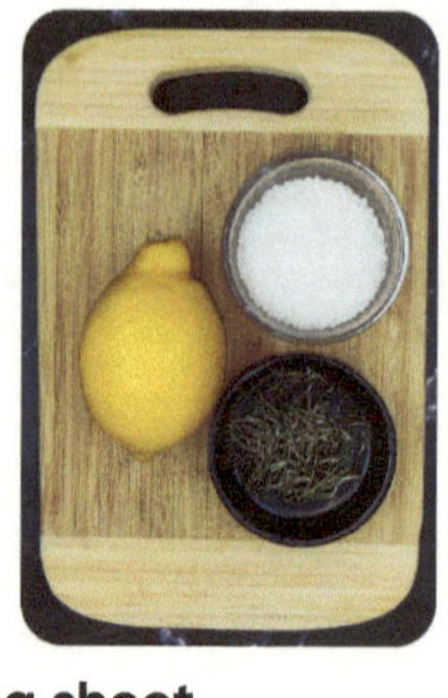

<u>Step 2 :</u>
- Spread the zest and rosemary on a baking sheet
- Put in the oven for 1 hour

<u>Step 3 :</u>
- Mix the salt, lemon zest and rosemary

<u>Step 4 :</u>
- Crush everything with the mortar

<u>Step 5 :</u>
- Put in an airtight container

<u>Ideal with:</u> fish and rice

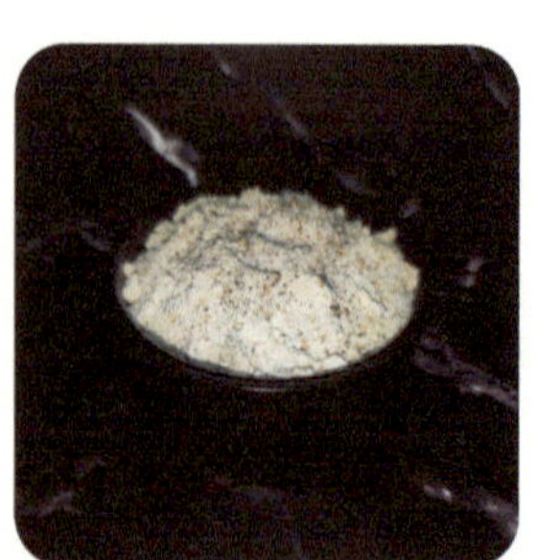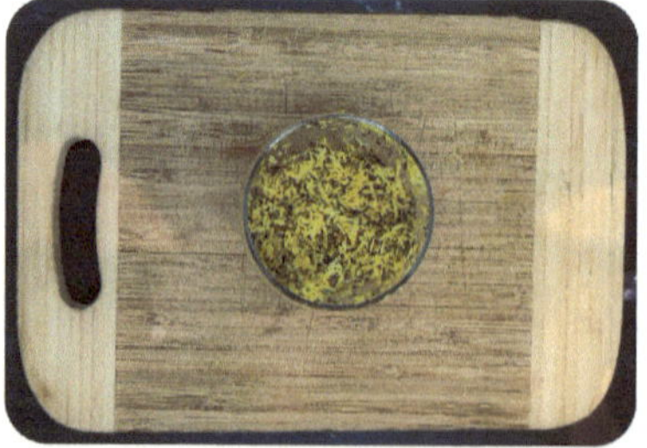

Salt/pepper

 **5min**

Ingrédients :
- **20g pepper**
- **80g fine salt**

Step 1 :
- **Mix everything**

Step 2 :
- **Put in an airtight container**

Ideal with: all dishes

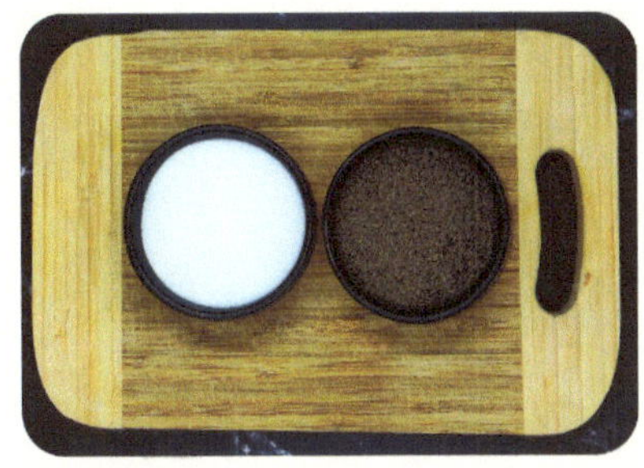

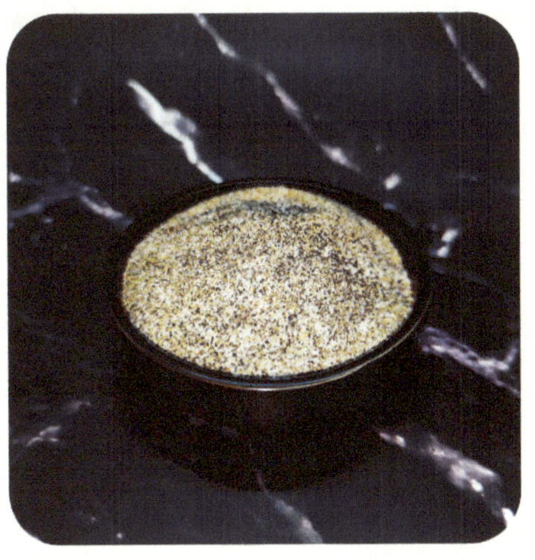

Scottish

 **45min**

<u>**Ingrédients :**</u>
- **5cl of whiskey**
- **100g salt**

<u>**Step 1 :**</u>
- **Preheat the oven to 90°C**
- **Mix everything**

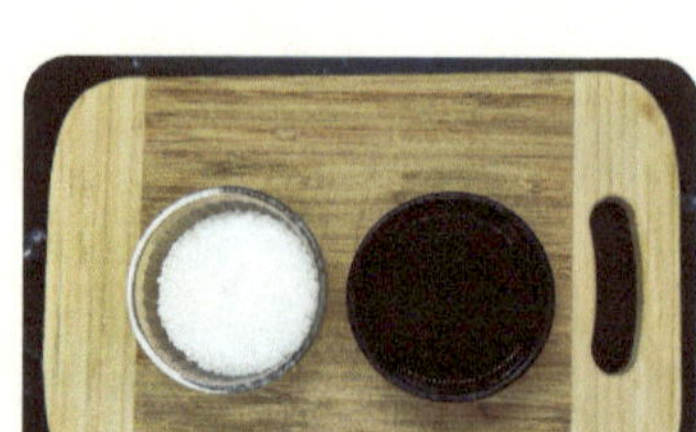

<u>**Step 2 :**</u>
- **Put on a baking sheet**
- **Put in the oven for 30 minutes**

<u>**Step 3 :**</u>
- **Put in an airtight container**

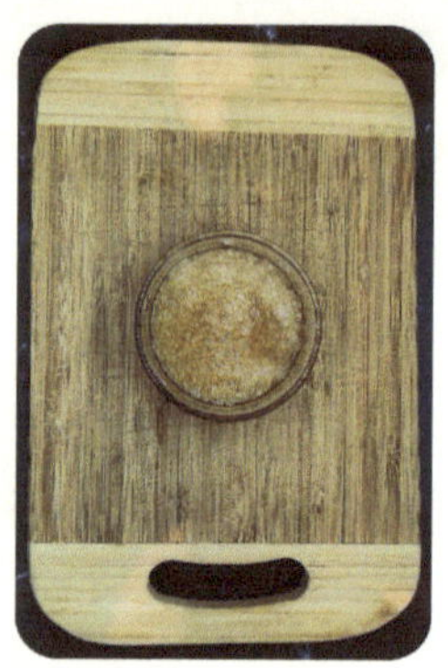

<u>**Ideal with:**</u> **meats and roasts**

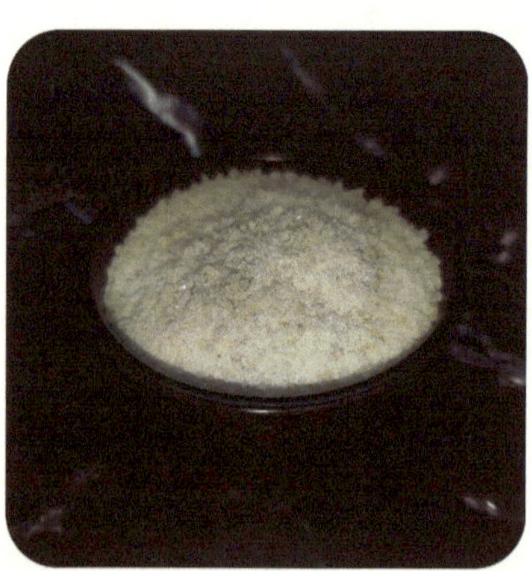

Smoked

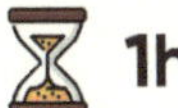 1h

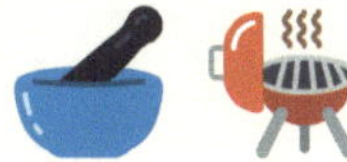

Ingrédients :
- 100g coarse salt

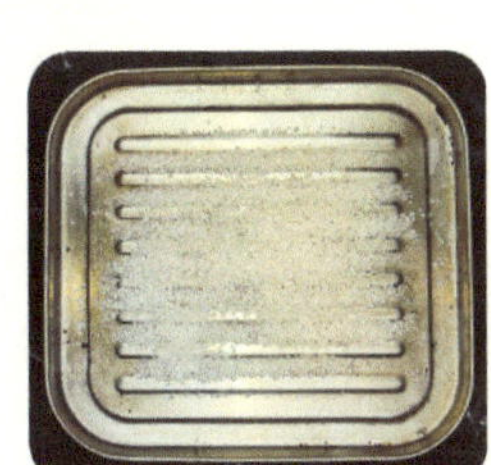

Step 1 :
- Lit the BBQ
- Wait until there are no more flames

Step 2 :
- Arrange the salt on a plate for the BBQ
- Put the plate on the BBQ
- Cover everything
- Leave to cook for 30 minutes

Option: You can put rosemary or other embers in the embers to flavor the salt

Step 3 :
- Crush everything with the mortar

Step 4 :
- Put in an airtight container

Ideal with: all dishes

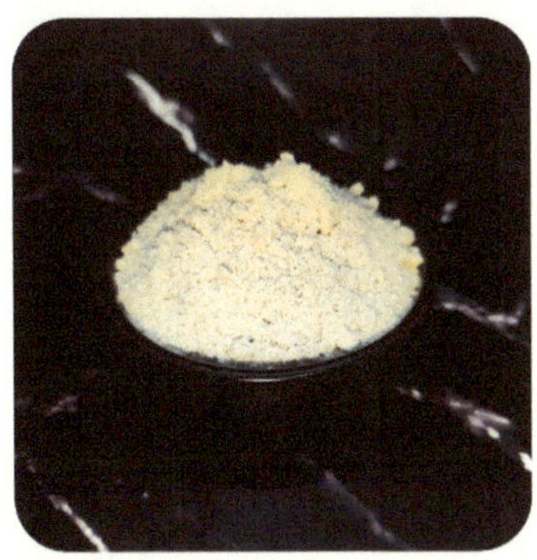

Vanilla

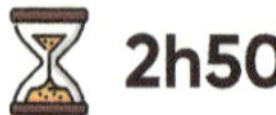

⏳ 2h50

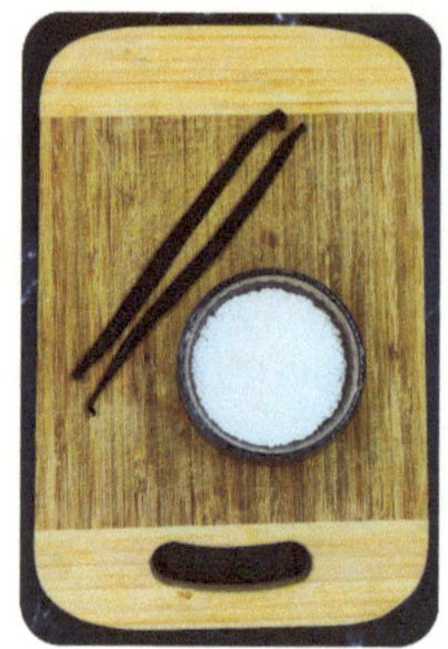

Ingrédients :
- 2 vanilla pods
- 100g salt

Step 1 :
- Mix the salt and vanilla
- Blend the salt and vanilla

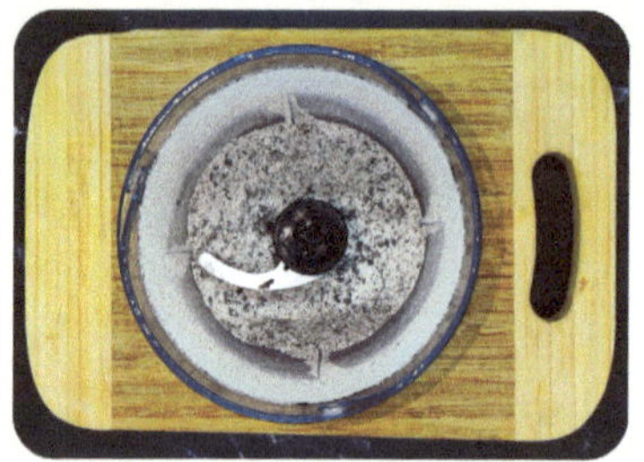

Step 2 :
- Put in an airtight container

Ideal with: fish and raw vegetables

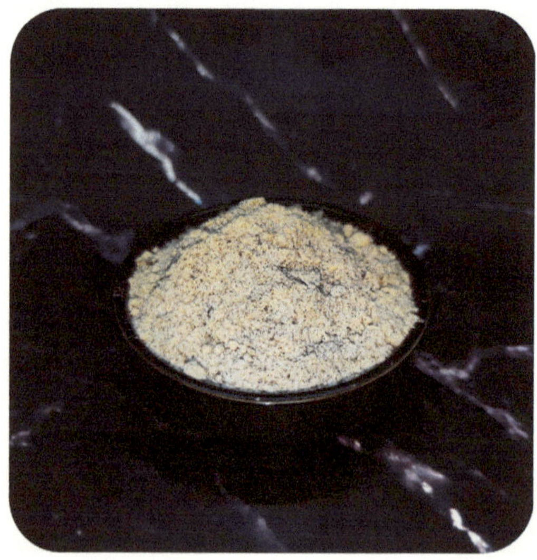

Vikings

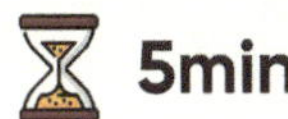 5min

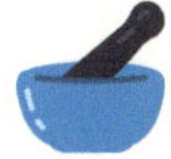

<u>Ingrédients :</u>
- 50g fine salt
- 20g grilled onion
- 8g cumin
- 7g of turmeric
- 7g of yellow mustard see
- 3g of fenugreek
- 2g coriander
- 1g of ginger
- 0.5g of black pepper

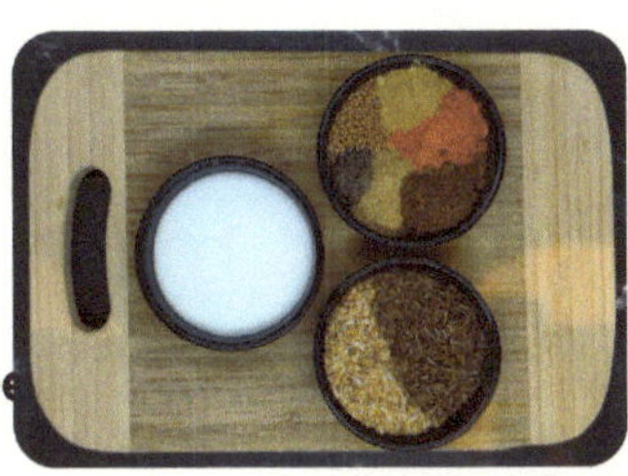

<u>Step 1 :</u>
- Mix all the ingredients

<u>Step 2 :</u>
- Crush everything in a mortar

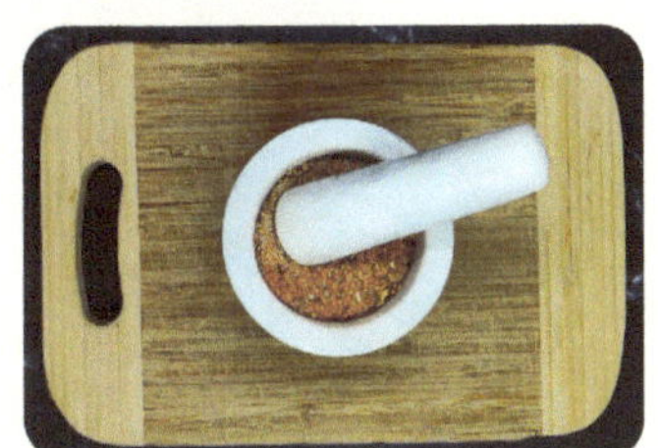

<u>Step 3 :</u>
- Put in an airtight container

<u>Ideal with:</u> **potato, egg and meat**

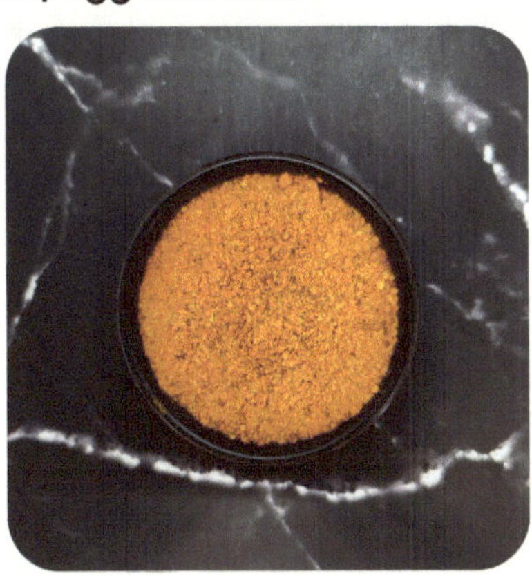

Wine

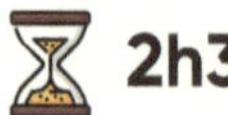 2h30

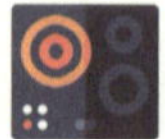 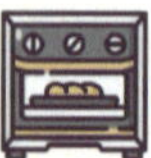 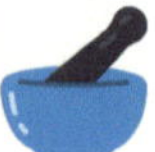

<u>Ingrédients :</u>
- 100g coarse salt
- 250-300cl of red wine

<u>Step 1 :</u>
- Preheat the oven to 90°C
- Bring the red wine to the boil
- Lower the heat
- Reduce over low heat until a smooth texture is obtained.

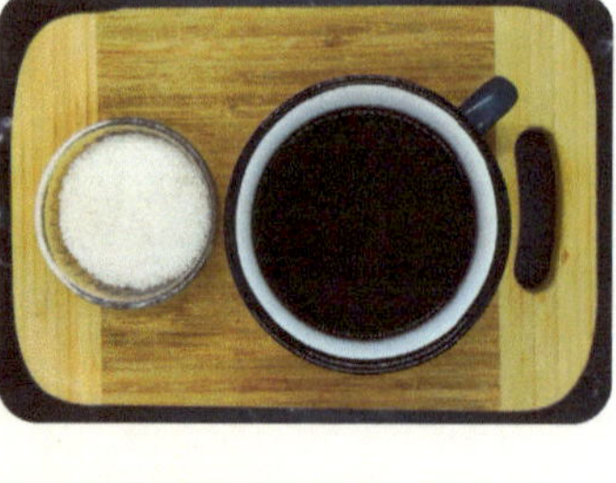

<u>Step 2 :</u>
- Mix the salt and the wine

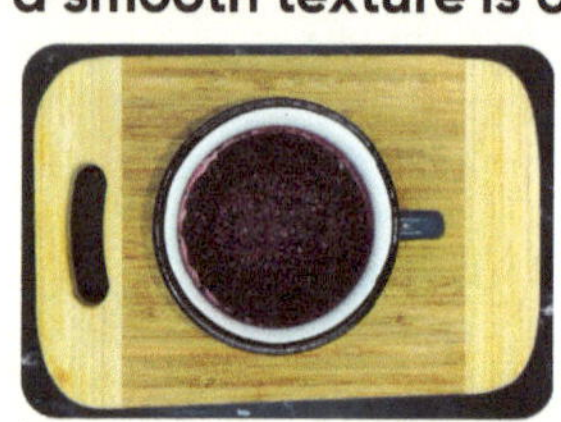

<u>Step 3 :</u>
- Spread the mixture on a baking sheet
- Put in the oven for 2 hours

<u>Step 4 :</u>
- Crush everything with the mortar

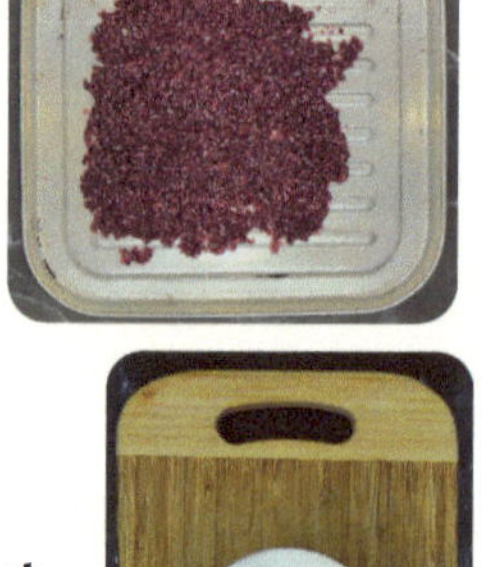

<u>Step 5 :</u>
- Put in an airtight container

<u>Ideal with:</u> red meat, duck and grilled meat

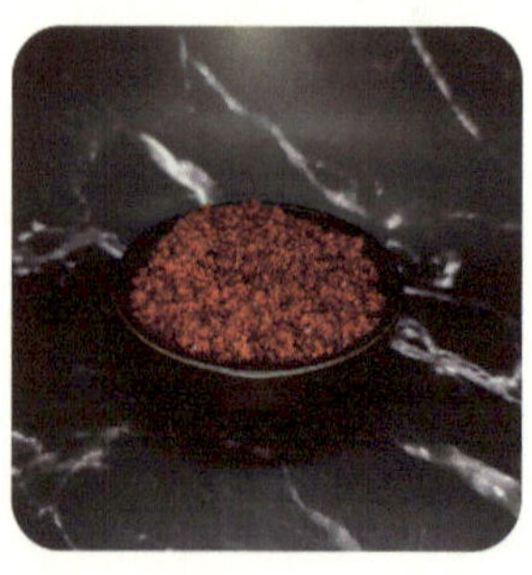

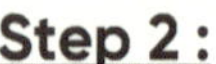
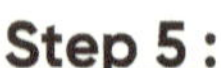
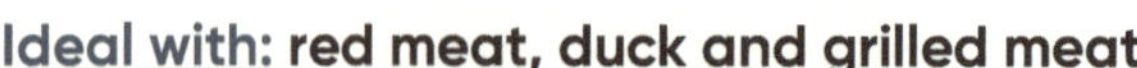

Who am I ? – Author

I am a generalist engineering school student who likes to cook, have fun and eat healthy.

So I started making my own homemade flavored salt recipes. Salts with more taste, nothing better.

As a result, sharing recipe ideas has become obvious.

The awareness of the quality of food impacting our health forced me to train in nutrition. So I did a nutrition certificate from Stanford.

In my childhood, I was able to learn to cook with my family and "manage" myself. Going through mistakes *(salt instead of sugar in a cake)* but you only learn by making mistakes. They allow us to improve so try to make recipes your way little by little and you will take even more taste in making them.

Mathis DAURIAT,

Acknowledgments

I would like to thank all of my family, relatives and friends for the various ideas and inspirations.

Thank you to my darling for being a tester *(of her own free will or not necessarily)* and for supporting me.

I also thank the readers for choosing this book and especially for having fun with homemade salt recipes with which they can now delight their friends and family!

Merci !

www.ingramcontent.com/pod-product-compliance
Lightning Source LLC
Chambersburg PA
CBHW041807260726
48664CB00035B/1442